ACTION PLAN FOR
DIABETES

ACTION PLAN FOR
DIABETES

DARRYL E. BARNES, MD

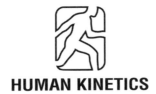

HUMAN KINETICS

Library of Congress Cataloging-in-Publication Data

Barnes, Darryl E.
   Action plan for diabetes / Darryl E. Barnes.
        p.   cm. -- (Action plan for health series)
   Includes bibliographical references and index.
   ISBN 0-7360-5459-6 (softcover)
   1. Diabetes. 2. Diabetes--Treatment. I. Title. II. Series.
   RC660.B285 2004
   616.4'6206--dc22

                                                                    2003021686

ISBN: 0-7360-5459-6

Copyright © 2004 by American College of Sports Medicine

Acquisitions Editor: Martin Barnard; **Developmental Editor:** Leigh LaHood; **Assistant Editor:** Carla Zych; **Copyeditor:** Jan Feeney; **Proofreader:** Sarah Wiseman; **Indexer:** Betty Frizzéll; **Permission Manager:** Toni Harte; **Graphic Designer:** Fred Starbird; **Graphic Artist:** Tara Welsch; **Photo Manager:** Dan Wendt; **Cover Designer:** Jack W. Davis; **Photographer:** Dan Wendt, unless otherwise noted; **Art Manager:** Kareema McLendon; **Illustrator:** Roberto Sabas; **Printer:** Versa Press

Human Kinetics books are available at special discounts for bulk purchase. Special editions or book excerpts can also be created to specification. For details, contact the Special Sales Manager at Human Kinetics.

Printed in the United States of America   10   9   8   7   6   5   4   3   2   1

Human Kinetics
Web site: www.HumanKinetics.com

United States: Human Kinetics
P.O. Box 5076
Champaign, IL 61825-5076
800-747-4457
e-mail: humank@hkusa.com

Canada: Human Kinetics
475 Devonshire Road Unit 100
Windsor, ON N8Y 2L5
800-465-7301 (in Canada only)
e-mail: orders@hkcanada.com

Europe: Human Kinetics
107 Bradford Road
Stanningley
Leeds LS28 6AT, United Kingdom
+44 (0) 113 255 5665
e-mail: hk@hkeurope.com

Australia: Human Kinetics
57A Price Avenue
Lower Mitcham, South Australia 5062
08 8277 1555
e-mail: liaw@hkaustralia.com

New Zealand: Human Kinetics
Division of Sports Distributors NZ Ltd.
P.O. Box 300 226 Albany
North Shore City
Auckland
0064 9 448 1207
e-mail: blairc@hknewz.com

This book is dedicated to my family and patients.

CONTENTS

ACKNOWLEDGMENTS

Thank you to Aimee, Kailee, Marlee, and Phoebe for allowing me the time to write this book, and to my patients for allowing me to learn from you all.

INTRODUCTION

Living with diabetes isn't easy. You know that diet and exercise are important in controlling your blood glucose, but how do you find balance in these areas without letting them take over your life? The answer lies in understanding how your body reacts to both diet and exercise and finding the practical solutions that allow you to enjoy your life and your health.

In most cases, exercise plays a pivotal role in diabetes prevention and is paramount in the treatment of this condition. But most important, exercise can play a major role in preventing complications associated with diabetes that can hinder your ability to thrive in your life.

I assume that you know that exercise can have positive effects on your health. In this book I introduce and discuss some practical tools that can help you plan an active and healthy lifestyle. Whether you are newly diagnosed with prediabetes, or whether you have had diabetes for a long time, I address questions that you may have about the specifics of starting and maintaining an exercise program, planning and following a healthy diet, and adjusting your medication based on your personal needs and goals.

Diabetes and the role of exercise in the treatment of this disease may seem complicated or confusing at first. Your physician may have told you that exercise is important but may be dangerous to your health if you do not plan your exercise, medication, and meals according to a specific schedule. Or maybe your doctor simply told you that you need to exercise more and eat less. Are these suggestions really solutions? For most of us, absolutely not. These types of suggestions are only introductions to solutions. You know how difficult, and sometimes even overwhelming, it can be if you do not have specific guidance in personal endeavors. What you really need is practical information on how to do these things. But in the current era of managed health care, most physicians have a difficult time delivering this information effectively in one office visit.

If these concerns are familiar to you, you're not alone. You'll start your action plan by understanding three basic principles. First, it is important to recognize the complications associated with diabetes. I explain how to recognize and deal with these problems, and why it is so important to do so early when exercising with diabetes. Second, you need to monitor your progress toward your goals and respond to change during this process. I explain how to monitor your eating habits, medication dosages, and exercise habits, and why this is essential to your success. Finally, you need to learn how to maintain control of your condition with exercise. I explain how to stay on track, even when distractions arise, and discuss why this will lead to lifelong success.

So what about those pounds you have been told to lose to prevent diabetes or optimize your diabetes treatment? Many studies have shown a close correlation between diabetes and obesity. In other words, most people with diabetes are overweight. Studies have also demonstrated that exercise can prevent or treat both diabetes and obesity. However, we all know how difficult losing weight can be—especially if the ultimate goal is to be thin. Fortunately, the data suggest that the amount of exercise required to treat obesity (to lose significant amounts of weight) is greater than that required to improve the condition of diabetes (controlling blood sugar levels). Your chances of success in minimizing diabetic complications are greater than your chances of fitting into the clothes you wore in high school. This means that you will likely see improvements in your diabetes before you realize a change in your physical appearance through weight loss. I describe ways to monitor your success in ways other than getting on the scale.

You are probably aware of the many methods of weight loss that have been described over the years. Weight-loss medications have been made available over the counter or by prescription. Many are available online or by mail. There have been a number of dieting methods available as well. You may have tried one or know someone who has. However, it is clear that pills or diets alone do not produce long-term success; nor do programs that incorporate exercise always work. Most of these weight-loss methods fail to produce long-term success because they do not address the principle of permanent lifestyle change, which involves healthy eating habits *and* exercise.

So what should you do when you are told that you have diabetes? The answer is not to just go out and find a diet plan or join the local gym. The simplest answer is to learn about your disease and how you can safely improve your specific condition by balancing your life with exercise. My commitment to you is to help you do just that. Once you understand your condition and what will improve it, only then can you make realistic, permanent changes that will allow you to enjoy a full and active life. So let's start your action plan for diabetes!

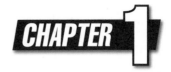
UNDERSTANDING DIABETES

You probably have an idea of what diabetes mellitus is, given that you are reading this book. But I have often found that many patients do not have an adequate grasp of their medical condition and thus have not been able to optimally participate in their own health care. So in this chapter I discuss the basics of diabetes.

Diabetes is a condition that affects more than 16 million Americans, of whom nearly one-third have yet to be diagnosed. Diabetes is characterized by elevated blood glucose, or sugar level (Harris et al. 1998). When a person without diabetes consumes food that contains carbohydrates, the main source for glucose in the blood, it is absorbed through the gastrointestinal tract and filters into the bloodstream. Once the sugar is in the blood, the body has a mechanism to recognize the level of blood sugar in the body. When a person eats, his blood sugar rises and the pancreas (an organ in the abdominal cavity) senses that the blood glucose level has risen and produces a substance called insulin. These cells in the pancreas allow glucose to flow through them via a special protein called GLUT-2 (glucose-transporter). When the glucose levels are higher than normal it is carried across GLUT-2 and starts a chain reaction that leads to the production of insulin, which is then released into the blood. You can think of insulin as the key to the door of the cell. When insulin is released from the pancreas into the blood, it comes in contact with cells in the peripheral tissues (muscle and fat); special pores (the doors) are unlocked, allowing glucose to flow into the cell, providing it with energy (see figure 1.1). The special doors in the peripheral tissues are made up of a special protein similar to those on the pancreas referred to as GLUT-4. This series of events is the mechanism that keeps the blood glucose at a normal level. In people with diabetes, the mechanism works abnormally. It is important to note that the brain and other cells have special proteins called GLUT-3 and GLUT-1 that are not dependent on insulin to function.

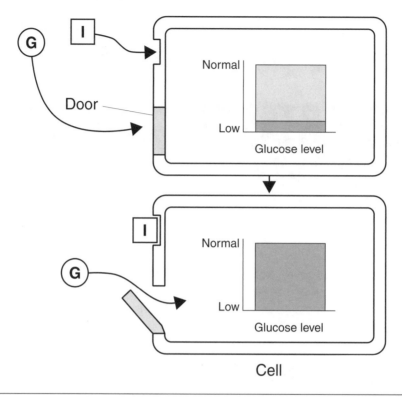

Figure 1.1 In a person without diabetes, insulin released from the pancreas acts as a key to open the cell door (GLUT-4) for glucose from the blood to enter.

Types of Diabetes

There are different types of diabetes, and the causes for the elevations in blood sugar differ depending on the type of diabetes you have. In this book I focus on the two major types of diabetes. The first form of diabetes that I'll discuss is called type 1 diabetes mellitus (or simply type 1 DM), sometimes referred to as insulin-dependent diabetes (IDDM), because people with this type of diabetes are reliant on an external source of insulin, which is injected. Type 1 DM is a condition in which the blood sugar levels are elevated because there is no production of insulin by the pancreas. In other words, these people do not produce the keys to the doors of the cell, and thus the glucose in the bloodstream cannot get into the cell (see figure 1.2a). These people have symptoms early in their lives, typically occurring in childhood or when they are young adults. Some people with type 1 diabetes may have inherited a susceptibility this condition. We think that in these people there is a reaction in the body that destroys insulin-producing cells in the pancreas, making it necessary for these people to take insulin in order to survive.

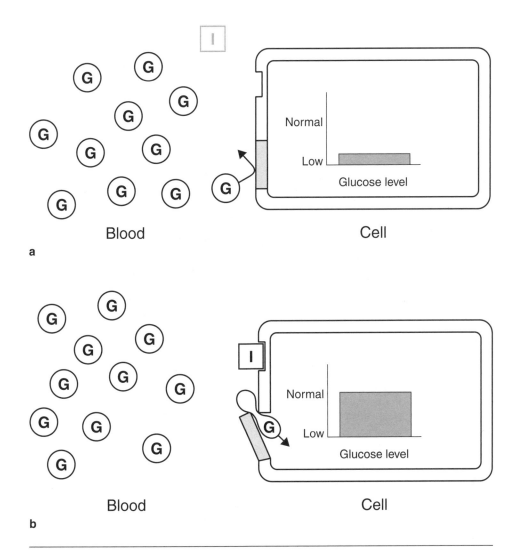

Figure 1.2 Two types of diabetes: *(a)* With type 1 diabetes, insulin is not present, so the glucose cannot get into the cell. *(b)* With type 2 diabetes, insulin is present, but the cell is less sensitive to it, so the glucose has a hard time getting into the cell.

The second type of diabetes is called type 2 diabetes mellitus (type 2 DM), sometimes referred to as non-insulin-dependent diabetes (NIDDM), because people with this type of diabetes typically do not need to take insulin (although some with type 2 diabetes will require insulin to control their glucose). This form of diabetes accounts for around 95 percent of people who have diabetes, and this form is the primary focus of this book. As in all cases of diabetes, those with type 2 have elevated blood glucose levels. However, unlike those with type 1, these people can produce insulin. Some even may produce more insulin than normal. The problem in this case has not much to do with the "key," insulin, but rather with the door's keyhole that allows it to open. If you have type 2 diabetes you have a high glucose level and either a low, normal, or high insulin level at the same time. The main problem in this case is that your cells are significantly less sensitive—or more resistant—to insulin and, in an attempt to keep the level of glucose inside the cells normal, the body creates a high concentration of glucose outside of the cells (see figure 1.2b). A type of diabetes similar to type 2 diabetes occurs during pregnancy, and I briefly discuss this later in this chapter. However, the information in this book is not intended as a comprehensive resource for those who are pregnant but only to give you a basic understanding of this condition.

Diagnosing Diabetes

Those with type 2 diabetes are usually diagnosed in their 30s. However, we are seeing more and more patients diagnosed in their teenage years. There may be a genetic predisposition, similar to that of type 1 diabetes, that may be linked to the development of type 2 diabetes. However, unlike those with type 1 diabetes, many people with type 2 diabetes (60 percent) are obese. This is likely due to a combination of genetic factors and may be a result of the body's need to take in more calories to keep blood sugar levels high enough for cells to function.

The common symptoms of type 1 and type 2 diabetes are similar and are directly related to the body's response to high blood sugar levels. The classic symptoms include excessive urination and thirst. When glucose is present in high levels in the blood, the kidneys produce higher volumes of urine. Thus, a person with untreated diabetes will have to empty the full bladder often. This can cause the body to become dehydrated, triggering the thirst response, resulting in excessive drinking. The volume of fluid that is lost in the urine is often great. And if this fluid is not replaced, the person can experience symptoms of dehydration as well, such as dizziness, headache, and rapid heart rate. Other symptoms include blurred vision, infections, and weight loss despite an increase in appetite and food consumption.

A major difference between type 1 and type 2 diabetes is that those with type 1 diabetes are absolutely dependent on an external source of insulin to live. These people may be presented with life-threatening symptoms. For example, if the person with type 1 diabetes does not have insulin, he will start to metabolize other energy sources in the body (such as fat) that produce harmful substances that can lead to death. This condition is called diabetic ketoacidosis (DKA). It is rare for someone with type 2 diabetes to develop DKA unless he is under very stressful conditions, such as a major illness.

Common Symptoms of Diabetes

- ▷ Excessive thirst
- ▷ Excessive urination
- ▷ Dehydration
- ▷ Dizziness
- ▷ Headache
- ▷ Rapid heart rate
- ▷ Blurred vision
- ▷ Infections*
- ▷ Weight loss*

*More commonly associated with type 1 diabetes mellitus.

The difference in body weight between those with type 1 and type 2 diabetes is commonly related to the effects insulin has on the body. Insulin supports growth of body tissues, including fat. People with type 1 diabetes, as discussed earlier, do not produce their own insulin, so they need to balance what they eat with the amount of insulin they take in order to keep their blood glucose levels normal. (I will discuss this more in chapter 5.) People with type 2 diabetes typically produce enough insulin and sometimes even two or three times the normal amount of insulin (DeFronzo 1988). In a person with untreated type 2 diabetes, the body senses that there is a low level of glucose inside the cells (despite having high levels in the blood), and the insulin level is increased and the hunger center in the brain is activated, driving the person to eat more. This combination of events often causes the person with type 2 diabetes to overeat, which leads to obesity.

Does everyone with diabetes have symptoms? Often there are symtoms. But just as often the diagnosis is made without the presence of symptoms, during routine health examinations that include blood sugar screenings. Elevated blood sugar prompts the health care provider to seek a cause of this irregularity. The physician may run more tests if an initial blood test is abnormal; she may review family history as well. We typically screen patients for diabetes starting at age 45. However, if a patient is in a high-risk group (African American, Asian, Latino, Native American) or has risk factors for diabetes (such as obesity, high blood pressure, high blood lipid levels, or a first-degree relative with diabetes), we screen the patient for diabetes earlier than age 45.

Risk Factors for Diabetes

▷ Member of a high-risk group (African American, Asian, Latino, Native American)

▷ Obesity

▷ High blood pressure

▷ High blood lipid levels

▷ First-degree relative with diabetes

Physicians prefer to have blood glucose tested in the morning, before the patient has eaten. This is called a fasting glucose test. We consider a normal fasting glucose test to be less than 110 mg/dl (milligrams per deciliter). If a person's fasting glucose level is between 110 and 126 mg/dl, then we consider this person to have prediabetes, or what is often referred to as glucose intolerance. Fasting glucose levels above 126 mg/dl on two separate occasions are indicative of diabetes mellitus. If you have a test after you have already eaten (or what is described as a nonfasting glucose test), and it shows your blood glucose level to be above 200 mg/dl, then this is enough to make the diagnosis of diabetes mellitus (see table 1.1).

There are other tests that may be done as well, such as a glucose tolerance test. The glucose tolerance test involves doing a fasting glucose test and then having the patient drink 75 milligrams of glucose and remeasuring the blood glucose levels after two hours. The test is normal if the fasting glucose is less than 110 mg/dl and the two-hour glucose level is less than 140 mg/dl. If the two-hour results show a level between 140 and 200 mg/dl, then this is indicative of glucose intolerance; up to 5 percent of patients with this level of blood glucose will develop diabetes. A two-hour glucose level greater than 200 mg/dl is indicative of diabetes.

Your doctor may also choose to do another test commonly referred to as the hemoglobin A_{1C} (HbA_{1C}). This is a test designed to give your health

Table 1.1 Glucose Levels and What They Mean

Diagnosis	Glucose level
Normal fasting glucose	<110 mg/dl
Prediabetes	110-126 mg/dl
Diabetes (2 separate measurements)	>126 mg/dl
Diabetes (nonfasting)	>200 mg/dl

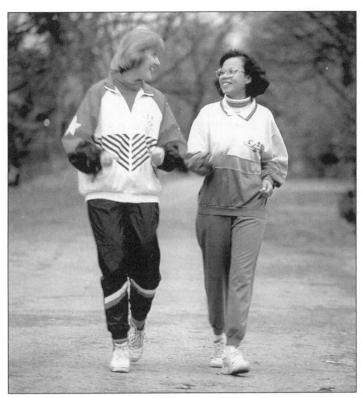

Although maintaining an exercise program may require some lifestyle changes, the benefits of exercise and its effects on your health are worth the work.

care provider a rough estimate of how high your blood glucose levels have been over the last three months. This can help your physician in deciding how often to check your glucose as well as in formulating your treatment plan. For instance, if your initial test confirms the diagnosis of type 2 diabetes with two fasting glucose levels of 130 mg/dl, that is just above the diagnostic threshold of 126 mg/dl. But if your HbA_{1c} is significantly elevated, your doctor may decide to monitor you more closely and treat your condition more aggressively. This may include starting a medication regimen earlier in addition to making changes in your diet and exercise habits. It is important to note that if you are diagnosed with type 1 diabetes, then you will start taking medication (insulin) immediately.

Other tests can differentiate between type 1 and type 2 diabetes if it becomes difficult to do through questioning the patient about symptoms. A certain molecule called C-peptide is part of the precursor molecule to the insulin molecule. When insulin is formed in the pancreas, the C-peptide separates from the insulin portion of the molecule and can be measured in the blood of those with type 2 diabetes, whereas it is not present in those with type 1 diabetes, because they do not produce insulin.

Gestational Diabetes

Gestational diabetes mellitus, or GDM, is similar to type 2 diabetes, but it diminishes after pregnancy. This condition occurs in up to 6 percent of women during pregnancy. If you have gestational diabetes or are pregnant and have type 2 diabetes, your health care team must monitor your condition closely. In addition, pregnancy may hinder your action plan if you are not aware of the potential problems. Those with type 1 diabetes who become pregnant need to be monitored exceptionally closely during pregnancy and should not start any new exercise or continue physical activities without explicit clearance by a physician experienced in the field of reproductive endocrinology. It is beyond the scope of this book to address the treatment or specific action plan of gestational diabetes or type 1 and type 2 diabetes during pregnancy. However, you should be aware of the important role exercise can play in the treatment of diabetes in pregnancy.

Pregnancy, especially in women with diabetes, alters glucose metabolism. Like type 2 diabetes, gestational diabetes is caused by insulin insensitivity or resistance. And just as it is in those with type 1 and type 2 diabetes, good glucose control is very important in those with gestational diabetes. But the condition for women with gestational diabetes is somewhat different than it is for women with type 2 who aren't pregnant. In gestational diabetes, glucose uptake by muscles and liver production of glucose is reduced even further (Artal 1996). In addition, the glucose demand of the fetus results in lower fasting blood glucose levels and increased blood glucose levels after meals because of insulin resistance. Most oral hypoglycemic agents are not used for treating gestational diabetes because they enter the placenta (the nutrient source for the fetus) and can adversely affect the fetus. However, some mothers with gestational diabetes take insulin to control their glucose levels. Insulin does not enter the placenta and thus does not directly affect the fetus. Nonetheless, hypoglycemia, the direct effect of too much insulin in the mother's blood, will adversely affect the fetus.

The fetus is entirely dependent on nutrition (carbohydrate, protein, fat, vitamins, and minerals) from its mother. Therefore, the fetus is at risk for hypoglycemia that the mother may experience if she has gestational diabetes, especially if she exercises or takes insulin to control her glucose levels. The risk of hypoglycemia is significant in a woman with gestational diabetes who is starting an exercise or insulin regimen. A physician who is experienced in treating women with gestational diabetes should monitor the condition closely.

Exercise and proper nutrition can play a pivotal role in treating gestational diabetes or type 2 diabetes in those who are pregnant, just as these measures can for those who are not pregnant (Artal 1996). When the diabetes health care team takes care of a pregnant patient, they take into consideration the decreased capacity for exercise caused by changes in anatomy and physiology. But the correct diagnosis needs to be made, because it is possible that hyperglycemia in pregnancy can be caused by the absence of insulin production (type 1 diabetes), which, if not diagnosed and treated early and properly, can result in severe complications for the mother and fetus such as poor fetal health, excess fetal growth that may interfere with vaginal delivery, and diabetic ketoacidosis.

Women who are physically active and then become pregnant are at lower risk of complications during pregnancy than those who start exercising after they become pregnant. This risk of a complication is amplified in those who already have diabetes or develop gestational diabetes. But the prime goal in relation to exercise should be glucose control. The generally accepted fasting glucose levels are between 95 and 105 mg/dl, and the after-meal glucose level is lower than 140 mg/dl at one hour and less than 120 mg/dl at two hours after meals. If glucose is not controlled with diet modification and exercise, then insulin treatment should be started (Turok 2003).

If you are pregnant or become pregnant, discuss your action plan for diabetes with your doctor before continuing with the action plan. Also be aware of the contraindications to exercise during pregnancy shown in table 1.2.

Table 1.2 Contraindications to Exercise During Pregnancy

Relative contraindications	Absolute contraindications
High blood pressure (hypertension)	History of 3 or more spontaneous abortions
Irregular heartbeat (arrhythmia)	Ruptured membrane (water breaks too early)
Anemia	Premature labor
Thyroid disease	Multiple gestation
Type 1 diabetes	Incompetent cervix
History of preterm labor	Bleeding or placenta previa
Bleeding during the current pregnancy	Restrictive lung disease
Fetus in the breech position (head up) during the last trimester	Symptomatic cardiac disease (moderate to severe)
Seizure disorder	Placental problems
Chronic bronchitis	Fetal distress
Orthopedic limitations	Fetal growth problems
Excessive obesity	Pregnancy-induced hypertension
Extreme underweight	Preeclampsia

Adapted, with permission from Artal R. Exercise: an alternative therapy for gestational diabetes. *Phys Sportsmed* 1996; 24(3):54-66. © 2004 The McGraw-Hill Companies.

Treatment Basics

At this point you should have a working knowledge of diabetes. It should be clear that those with diabetes are characterized as having abnormally high blood glucose levels and that there are different forms of diabetes. The main difference between type 1 and type 2 diabetes is in the treatment: People with type 1 diabetes require treatment with an external source of insulin, and those with type 2 diabetes are typically treated initially with a modification of their diet and exercise habits because exercise can make the body more sensitive to insulin (Devlin 1992). However, some people with type 2 may require medication to help them produce more insulin or to make them more sensitive to it (see table 1.3). Some with type 2 may even require injections of insulin to control their glucose levels. Using exercise as a treatment for type 2 diabetes is the focus of this book. I discuss important issues concerning the use of exercise in the treatment of type 1 diabetes as well.

The main goal of treating diabetes is to prevent complications of the disease. Many studies have shown that keeping the blood glucose at normal levels can be effective in eliminating the symptoms and slowing or preventing the potentially devastating complications associated with diabetes. We will discuss these complications in more detail in the following chapters.

How many times have you heard someone say, "Just eat right and exercise"? If it were as easy as it sounds, type 2 diabetes would not be nearly as common as it is. But eating right and exercising are not easy. Most of us do not even understand what "eating right" is. Our society inundates us with advertisements that encourage us to eat more. When was the last time that you were at a fast-food drive-up window and the attendant asked you if you'd like to *decrease* the size of your value meal?

Table 1.3 Treatment of Type 1 and Type 2 Diabetes

Treatment	Type 1 diabetes	Type 2 diabetes
Insulin	Yes (all)	Yes (rare)
Hypoglycemic agents	No	Yes (common)
Exercise	Yes (reduces complications but does not treat diabetes)	Yes
Healthy diet	Yes (reduces complications but does not treat diabetes)	Yes

The most common excuse that I hear is, "I do not have time to exercise." Typically, this response comes from a person who does not understand how useful exercise can be in treating the condition. It is well known that exercise can improve almost anyone's health. People who have type 1 diabetes can benefit from exercise as well. But for someone with type 2 diabetes, exercise is a major component of treatment and in many cases may prevent the disease. The addition of physical activity to your life may be the only treatment you need for your diabetes.

You now have a good foundation of knowledge about your disease, which will help you understand the steps to creating your action plan for healthful living.

ACTION PLAN:

UNDERSTANDING DIABETES

☐ Become familiar with what actually goes on in the bloodstream and cells of a person with type 1 or type 2 diabetes.

☐ Learn about the diagnosis and risk factors of the disease.

☐ Understand that you have the power to prevent complications of diabetes through developing an action plan that includes regular exercise and healthful eating habits.

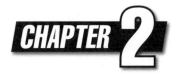
MAKING GLUCOSE CONTROL YOUR GOAL

Many scientific studies show that the most effective way to decrease or eliminate the complications associated with diabetes is to keep blood glucose at or near normal levels. Most health problems that are associated with diabetes arise without many symptoms. Not knowing this simple fact can be a major roadblock to living a healthy life. If you don't know that a threat to your life exists, then how can you attempt to prevent it? Say you have 45,000 miles on your car and you want to drive your car 20 miles down a steep canyon. Tucked away in the glove box is the manual that states that the braking system should be serviced at 40,000 miles to prevent its potential failure. And say that you did not happen to read every page of your car's manual and did not know this particular fact. You would likely drive down the canyon completely unaware of the potential danger that lies ahead. Likewise, if glucose control is not your goal, potential dangers lie ahead. In this chapter we discuss the complications of poorly controlled diabetes.

The visual system (eyes), renal system (kidneys), cardiovascular system (heart), peripheral vascular system (blood vessels in the extremities), nervous system (nerves), gastrointestinal system (stomach and intestines), and immune system (infection control) are the bodily systems affected by poor diabetes control. Given that many of these systems interrelate, I discuss diabetes as it relates to vision, the kidneys, the heart and blood vessels, and the nervous system. The effects on gastrointestinal and immune system are discussed as well. These complications are summarized in table 2.1.

Table 2.1   Systems Affected by Diabetes

Organ system	Common signs and symptoms
Ocular system (eyes)	Blurred vision, blindness
Renal system (kidneys, bladder)	Protein wasting in urine, high blood pressure, urinary tract infections
Cardiovascular system (heart)	Coronary artery disease, heart attack
Peripheral vascular system (blood vessels of the arms and legs)	Leg and foot pain with activity, skin and soft-tissue breakdown
Central nervous system (brain)	Stroke or cerebral vascular incident
Peripheral nervous system (nerves in the torso, arms, and legs)	Foot numbness and pain, foot ulcers, nausea, vomiting, diarrhea, loss of bladder control, light-headedness, loss of consciousness
Immune system (infection-control system)	Frequent infections (skin and bladder infections are common)

Diabetes and Your Vision

Diabetes is a leading cause of blindness in the United States, and the best means of early detection of vision problems is to have an ophthalmologist examine your eyes by dilating them and observing the retina. It is recommended that all people with type 1 diabetes have annual eye exams starting five years after the onset of their condition. Those with type 2 diabetes should have an examination soon after their diagnosis is made. Any visual changes that occur should be taken seriously; such changes warrant a complete eye exam by an ophthalmologist.

Diabetes affects the eyes by damaging the retina, which is referred to as diabetic retinopathy. The retina is the part of the eye that is responsible for sensing light. Retinal damage can occur in two ways. First, the blood vessels that supply nutrients to the cells of the retina can become damaged as a consequence of high glucose levels in the blood that in turn cause bleeding and the formation of blood clots in them. The blood from these vessels that leaks into the eye can obscure light from reaching the retina, causing blindness. And if the retina cannot receive nutrients and oxygen because of a lack of blood flow in the vessels, the cells will die, causing permanent loss of vision.

Sometimes when small blood vessels in the retina are damaged in this way the body will produce new vessels in this area to try to deliver oxygen to the retinal cells. This can lead to far too many new blood vessels being formed in the retina, which in turn block out light and cause blindness. This condition is called proliferative diabetic retinopathy. The current treatment of this condition involves the use of a special laser to slow or stop new vessel overgrowth.

Blurring of vision can also occur when the blood glucose is high. These symptoms can sometimes be resolved when the blood glucose is brought under control. However, it is also known that high glucose levels can lead to nerve damage that can affect the way your eye moves. This is often a permanent condition. If the nerves to your eye muscles do not work properly, blurring of vision will occur.

Diabetes and Your Kidneys

According to the American Diabetes Association, 10 to 21 percent of people with diabetes have kidney disease, referred to as diabetic nephropathy. The kidneys are organs that filter out unnecessary products from your bloodstream and retain the necessary elements, such as proteins and electrolytes (sodium and potassium). However, high glucose levels can lead to an abnormality that allows necessary elements in your blood, such as proteins, to be wasted into the urine. This is referred to as proteiuria, which is a common sign of early kidney failure. Good glucose control through proper diet, exercise, and medication if needed can prevent diabetic nephropathy (Hostetter 2003).

Damage to your kidneys can also lead to the development of high blood pressure, also called hypertension. If you develop high blood pressure, it is important that you control your blood pressure. But if you develop high blood pressure and you have diabetes, it is even more important for you to control your blood pressure. The diseases that are directly related to high blood pressure, such as heart, eye, and kidney disease, may progress more rapidly in someone with diabetes and high blood pressure. Some classes of blood pressure–lowering medications may be more beneficial than others for diabetics with kidney problems. Your physician will need to take into account your medical condition to determine what medications are best for you.

Further damage to the kidneys can occur from untreated or under-treated urinary tract infections. Infections of the bladder are often controlled easily with the implementation of antibiotics. People with diabetes are more susceptible to these types of infections and at a greater risk of kidney damage if the infection spreads from the bladder to the kidneys causing them to become infected, too. This type of infection is commonly referred to as pyelonephritis.

It is also important that diabetics with kidney problems not receive contrast materials (a substance that is typically used when your doctor

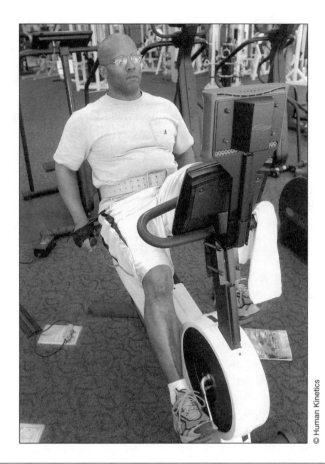

© Human Kinetics

Controlling glucose through exercise is one key to preventing other health problems that can result from diabetes.

orders special X rays) in their blood until receiving clearance from physicians. We know that these contrast agents can cause kidney damage in anyone, but we also know that those with diabetes are at an increased risk for this to occur. You should carry a medical alert card or something similar to identify you as a person with diabetes in case you require emergency treatment that involves contrast materials. A medical alert card, bracelet, or necklace will allow the medical team to take appropriate steps to protect you from potential harm.

Your doctor can monitor your kidney functioning by using lab tests, which include urine tests for glucose and protein. If your blood glucose is greater than 180 mg/dl, then glucose will appear in your urine; a urine test for elevated glucose levels can be helpful if blood glucose readings are unavailable. In fact, this is how many people with diabetes are initially diagnosed. As described previously, protein in the urine is usually indicative of kidney disease. Various methods of testing for protein in the urine include diagnostic test strips that are dipped into the urine and compared to standard colorimetric charts to determine estimated levels of substances including glucose and protein. This type of test is easy to use in the doctor's office, takes little time to complete, and is relatively inexpensive. Another test, called the 24-hour urine test, is more accurate and gives more specific levels of protein in the urine. Your doctor will typically order this test if your dip strip test is positive. If your 24-hour urine test shows that there are more than 30 milligrams of protein (albumin), your kidneys are having trouble retaining needed protein, which is evidence that damage has taken place in the kidneys. If this is the case, then your doctor may choose to place you on a common blood pressure medication known as an ACE inhibitor or angiotensin receptor II antagonist, even if you have normal blood pressure. Studies have shown that this particular drug not only controls blood pressure but also protects the kidneys in those with diabetes.

Diabetes and Your Cardiovascular System

Those with diabetes are at high risk for heart and vascular disease. The heart is a muscle that pumps blood throughout the body to supply it with nutrients and oxygen and to take away by-products of metabolism, such as carbon dioxide. Compared to other muscles in the body, the heart consumes a high amount of nutrients and oxygen. It pumps blood to itself through specialized vessels called coronary arteries. These arteries are critical to the integrity of the functioning of the heart. We know that diabetes can cause harm to these vessels, called coronary artery disease. This disease can be in the form of thickening of the vessels that can cause decreased blood flow through the vessel or the formation of fatty material, commonly referred to as a plaque, that blocks the flow of blood through the vessel. Both of these conditions can lead to a decreased or arrested blood flow to the heart, which will cause severe impairment to this pumping muscle. This is referred to as a myocardial infarction, or heart attack.

Similar problems can occur in larger vessels in the body, such as those leading to your arms and legs. Problems such as these are classified as peripheral vascular disease. With this condition, the blood vessels leading to the arms and legs can be impaired by thickening of the walls of the vessels or development of fatty plaque on the inside of the vessels. Peripheral vascular disease can lead to decreased blood flow to the limbs, causing pain and changes in the tissues. This tissue damage can lead to infections. Pain is a common complaint when the blood flow is decreased to most tissues in the body. Sometimes this will occur during activities when the muscles require increased oxygen. For instance, you may have vascular disease, causing a decreased blood flow to your extremities. When you are at rest you may not have pain because the flow is good enough for muscles to function. But when you start walking, activating your muscles, the oxygen demand is greater than the flow of blood allows, causing pain in the leg muscles. If you develop any problems like this, your doctor will order a test to assess the blood flow in your vessels in the affected limb. This is typically done with a machine that uses ultrasonic waves to measure flow in a blood vessel. Other tests can measure the amount of oxygen in the blood that is flowing, which can provide information helpful to determining the health of the limb.

The results can be devastating when the vessels that are diseased are in the brain. The brain requires oxygen at all times. Even a short period of oxygen deprivation can cause significant damage, which is often irreversible. This condition is commonly referred to as a stroke, or a cerebrovascular accident. The carotid arteries in the neck that supply your brain with oxygenated blood can become diseased (called carotid artery disease) thus decreasing blood flow, which can result in a stroke. If your physician suspects you may be at risk for a stroke, he may order an ultrasound test similar to that used to assess blood flow in the arms or legs.

It is well known that all people with diabetes have an increased risk of infections. This risk is further increased with the presence of vascular disease. The body's immune system consists of specialized cells that identify and destroy invading organisms. But when the blood flow that carries these cells to their destination is decreased, the ability of the cells to function normally is also decreased, leading to increased rates of infection.

Diabetes and Your Nervous System

In people with diabetes, the nervous system can be affected in many ways, causing multiple problems termed neuropathy. These problems can include numbness of sensation, increased pain sensation, decreased muscle control and function, and difficulty with control of other organs such as the bladder and bowel. There can also be significant problems with neurological control of the heart and blood vessels, which can lead to abnormal heart rhythms and significant fluctuations in blood pressure.

Those with diabetes who have decreased sensation can develop problems relating to the inability to sense pressure pain. For instance, if the soles of your feet do not sense pressure well, it will be difficult for you to know whether or not your shoe fits well. Therefore, when there is a specific pressure point on a part of your foot that you cannot feel, it will lead to significant breakdown of the skin, causing an ulcer that can become infected. This condition is called peripheral neuropathy; it is theorized that is directly caused by the by-products of hyperglycemia.

A decrease in sensation can also lead to a significant breakdown of joints, which in turn can lead to fractures and deformities. For example, if you moved a certain way that caused pain in your foot, you would investigate the cause and come up with the solution to stop the pain. But if you don't have the ability to sense this pain (the body's early warning system), you won't notice the damage until a visible change occurs. Such a change may be anything from swelling and redness to a drop in your arch, causing a large deformity of your foot. Foot care is very important for all people with diabetes. Your doctor can order a test called an electromyelogram (EMG) to look at your peripheral nerve function and health.

Damage to the nerves that control certain body parts can occur, resulting in dysfunction of the specific areas. This is referred to as autonomic neuropathy. These areas can include organs such as muscles, heart, blood vessels, stomach, intestine, and bladder. For example, if the nerves to your hand muscles were damaged, you may notice that you have decreased ability to manipulate small objects such as writing utensils. Similarly, if the nerves that control gastric motility (which is required for normal food digestion) are damaged, you may experience symptoms ranging from nausea and vomiting to constipation or diarrhea.

Furthermore, if the nervous system's interaction with the blood vessels is disrupted, this can result in the inability to control your blood pressure. The body's blood pressure normally is lower while lying or sitting than when standing. The nervous system helps increase the blood pressure when we go to the standing position. If your nervous system is impaired from diabetes, you may notice symptoms such as light-headedness, dizziness, or even loss of consciousness when you attempt to go from a lying or sitting position to a standing position. More importantly, normal autonomic nerve function is critical to exercising safely. I will discuss this more in chapter 4.

Caring for Your Feet

Foot problems are common in those with diabetes because uncontrolled diabetes can cause poor circulation, leading to nerve damage. You need to start caring for your feet as soon as possible to prevent or significantly delay many foot problems. Not making foot care a priority only puts you at greater risk for serious problems, including amputation. If you currently have foot problems, you should see a doctor experienced in foot care, such as a podiatrist, to ensure that you are incorporating the best care possible for your feet.

Foot Exams

Your action plan should include daily foot exams. As with all planning, try to find a time of day when you will most likely have the time and will remember to do this task. Many people find it easiest to do their foot checks just after getting ready for bed. You, or someone else if you are unable, will need to carefully inspect your feet. If you are doing this for yourself, then it will be helpful to use a mirror to look at those areas that are difficult to see.

When looking at your feet, be sure that you have adequate lighting so that you don't miss anything. Find a safe place to sit while doing the inspecting. Your goal during these sessions is to detect any evidence of skin lesions such as sores, scratches or cuts, swollen or red areas, calluses, corns, or any problem with your nails (such as ingrown or infected toenails). Look at all parts of your feet from the ankle down, including between each toe. Remember that you may not be able to feel some of the subtle pain that is typically associated with these foot problems. Report all cuts and scratches that do not start healing after 24 hours of discovery, or any painful, red, or warm areas to your physician immediately.

Foot Hygiene

Good hygiene is important in preventing foot problems. You should wash your feet each day. You may want to get a foot tub to clean your feet before you start the inspection process. Use warm (90 to 95 degrees Fahrenheit) rather than hot water, and use nondrying soap to clean your feet thoroughly. Do not soak your feet in water because this can wash away essential skin oils that give your feet natural protection. Dry skin will crack, and any openings in the skin can let bacteria and viruses in, causing infection. When you are finished washing your feet, rinse the soap off and thoroughly dry your feet with a clean and dry towel, being sure to dry between each toe. To ensure that your skin does not become overdry, apply a moisturizing cream or lotion to the tops and soles of your feet, gently rubbing it in and avoiding the areas between your toes. Lotion between your toes can lead to excessive moisture and cause the skin to break down, which may lead to an infection. Many people use talcum power to ensure that the areas between the toes stay dry.

After washing and inspecting your feet, trim your nails straight across to ensure that the edges do not become ingrown in the sides of the toes. If your nails are thick, you should have a podiatrist trim them for you. Before taking care of any corns or calluses (excess thick skin often found on the heel area), ask your podiatrist how you can do this at home. Using a pumice stone while your skin is still moist is helpful to gently smooth excess skin on your heels as well as calluses and corns. Avoid using over-the-counter chemical products to treat your calluses or corns, or using sharp instruments such as scissors, scalpels, or razor blades unless instructed by your doctor. These types of treatments may damage your skin, which can lead to infection.

If you find that you have calluses or corns on your heels and toes, this may be evidence of improper footwear. It is very important that your socks and shoes fit your feet well. Socks without thick seams or those that are seamless are better for your feet. Shoes that offer a wide toe box, smooth liners, good support, and breathable materials will be best for your feet. Vinyl and plastic are not good materials for shoes because they do not allow your feet to breathe. Furthermore, you should not wear shoes without socks because they will allow your foot to sweat and become too moist, which can lead to skin breakdown. Your socks offer extra protection from friction that your skin encounters inside a shoe, which will prevent blisters and cuts. Because of the increased risk of cuts, you should avoid going barefoot, especially in places where there may be broken glass such as in parks or at the beach.

Foot Protection

Protect your feet from the heat and the cold. Allowing your feet to become cold will decrease the sensation in them. In cold climates, wear thicker socks and shoes or boots that are lined with soft insulation. In addition, good blood circulation is important in keeping your feet warm. Avoid wearing tight socks or shoes and crossing your legs or standing in one place for extended periods. Especially avoid smoking tobacco because it decreases blood flow, resulting in cold feet. Protecting your feet from heat

Foot Care Basics

▷ Start your foot care plan now and make it a priority.

▷ Be sure to conduct a daily foot check.

▷ Have someone else check your feet if you are unable to do so yourself.

▷ Use a mirror to help you see those areas that are difficult to see.

▷ Check your feet in a well-lit room to make sure you can see any potential problems.

▷ Look for sores, scratches or cuts, swollen or red areas, calluses, and corn or nail problems.

▷ Remember to look between your toes.

▷ Tell your physician about all cuts that do not start to heal within 24 hours and all painful, red, or warm areas.

▷ Wash your feet every day with warm water and a nondrying soap.

▷ Do not soak your feet in water.

▷ Use a moisturizing cream or lotion on your feet. Avoid putting lotion between the toes.

▷ Trim your nails straight across to avoid ingrown nails.

▷ Always wear socks with shoes.

▷ Choose shoes with a wide toe box, smooth liners, good support, and breathable materials (cotton or leather).

▷ Avoid going barefoot.

▷ Protect your feet from excessive heat and cold.

▷ Don't smoke.

is just as important as protecting them from the cold. Avoid walking barefoot on heated surfaces such as hot asphalt or concrete. And remember to protect your skin by using sunscreen on your feet as well as on other exposed areas when you're in the sun.

Being proactive by doing foot checks before you encounter a problem is the most important part of good foot care. Talk with your health care team after you come up with a plan for the care of your feet to ensure that you have covered all of your bases. To find more information on foot care, visit www.ndep.nih.gov (a Web site of the National Institutes of Health) and www.diabetes.org (a Web site of the American Diabetes Association), or do a search online for diabetic foot care.

Glucose Control

I realize that you may be very uneasy after reading this chapter. Do all people with diabetes get all of these problems? The simple answer is no. However, you are at greater risk of having these complications. I think the better question would be whether you can prevent diabetes from causing these problems. The scientific data suggest that with good glucose control, most if not all of these complications can be prevented or minimized. For some, glucose control may be as easy as starting an exercise program. But some of you may require initiation in an exercise program, diet modifications, and medications under the close supervision of your physician. No matter where you fall in the range of patients, you can develop an action plan to control your glucose.

ACTION PLAN:
MAKING GLUCOSE CONTROL YOUR GOAL

☐ Understand the effects of diabetes on various bodily systems:

- Vision
- Kidneys
- Cardiovascular system
- Nervous system

☐ Listen to your body and talk to your doctor about any suspicions you may have in any of these areas.

☐ Make it your goal to control your glucose as a means of preventing further health problems.

☐ Remember that good foot care can prevent significant health problems.

CHAPTER 3

PLANNING YOUR LIFESTYLE

You may already have a plan that allows you to live with diabetes. But it's likely that you're reading this book to find a better way to improve and enjoy your health. It is no secret that planning ahead for any endeavor is crucial for success.

Lifestyle is a personal matter. It represents who you are, what you believe in, and what stage of life you are in. So why should you make plans for a new lifestyle? You already know why glucose control should be your goal. You also know that exercise needs to be a part of the process in obtaining the goal. So why don't you just go on a diet, start an exercise program, lose weight, and control your glucose? I'm sure you already know the answer: It's easier said than done! To do all of these things, you must make your own plans in your life that will lead to accomplishing your goal.

Understanding the process of what you need to do to accomplish a goal is paramount. For example, say you are the lead planner on a project for a spaceship company. This project's main goal is to send humans and several tons of cargo to Mars and safely return the people to Earth. Before you actually start to write anything down on paper, you would first think about what you were asked to do. You may consider your qualifications in taking on such an endeavor. You'd concern yourself with whether you had the right resources to take on such a project. This initial process will happen in your mind in a matter of seconds after receiving this task. You will then move on to the second process of organizing a team to help you gather the information to make this endeavor a success. Once you've completed the research and gathered the information, you will create a rough draft of a plan to get from Earth to Mars and back. From here, the process of refining the plan occurs, taking thousands of hours, millions of calculations, and hundreds of changes to the plan until the final process of putting the plan into action occurs.

Obviously, creating a lifestyle plan to thrive with diabetes is not nearly as complicated as the plan I just described. I used this example to illustrate the point that planning takes many steps to complete. As in the example, your initial process when you discovered you have diabetes took only seconds. When your doctor told you that your glucose was elevated and that you needed to control it, your immediate thoughts probably were *How can I do that?* or *Can you help me?* Your second process of organizing resources and gathering information started when you inquired about what you can do about your diabetes. Your "team" includes you, your health care providers, and your family and friends (see table 3.1). The information-gathering and research process is currently under way—you're reading this book.

In this chapter I give you the information you need to create a rough plan, a guide to assist you in making personal changes to create a lifestyle conducive to attaining your goals for glucose control through healthy living. The following chapters show you how to refine it until it works for you.

But even before we can create a plan for your new lifestyle, you need to consider the type of lifestyle you have now. Do you have an active lifestyle? What kind of exercise do you do? Can you control your eating habits? Do you feel like food controls you? Is your current lifestyle meeting your life's goals? Only you can answer these questions. You may already be active with healthy eating habits, but you'd like to know what you can do to optimize your action plan. But if you recognize that you do not have the lifestyle you would like or need, this chapter will help you most.

Table 3.1   Health Care Team

Health care team	Role
Physician	Coordinates and provides continuity of care for all medical problems. Assists in creating and modifying action plan.
Diabetes nurse educator	Provides resources and teaches people with diabetes how to treat themselves. Teaches how to use and maintain medical devices such as glucose monitors and injectable insulin devices (syringes, needles, pumps). Can help physician make decisions on insulin adjustments.
Dietitian	Provides guidance by helping patients select enjoyable meal plans that support health goals.

Your Current Lifestyle

As I mentioned previously, lifestyle is representative of the choices that you make. So in creating an action plan for diabetes, you must be able to go through the many processes of making healthy choices that will last throughout your lifetime. Honesty is key here. If you know that overeating is your major fault, then admit this to yourself. Do you hate to exercise, or think that you would not enjoy it? Do you know anyone who exercises? These are the types of questions you should ask yourself.

I have created a lifestyle-assessment form (see figure 3.1) that can help you work through this process and identify potential barriers to attaining your ideal lifestyle. There are no right or wrong answers; it is designed to get you to think about your current lifestyle while creating your action plan. A good way to use this form is to fill out the questionnaire portion now, then keep a daily log for two weeks. Then look back at your answers to see whether they correlate to what you thought. By then you will have read this entire book and discovered better ways to eat and exercise, and you'll be able to apply it to your lifestyle.

This is the initial process, such as when the lead planner in the space-ship project thought about her qualifications in taking on such a large endeavor. Ask yourself about your own qualifications to understand what your challenges will be in creating your action plan for diabetes. Start with

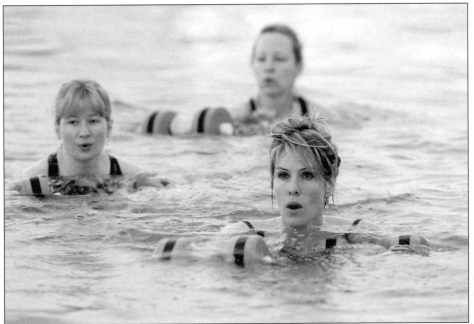

The accountability that comes from joining an exercise class, such as water aerobics, can help you stay on track with your own program.

LIFESTYLE ASSESSMENT FORM

Exercise

Do I currently do any form of exercise? _____

_____

If so, what exercise(s)? _____

_____

How often? _____

_____

What kinds do I enjoy most? _____

_____

Do I reward myself (other than with food) for exercising? _____

_____

Do I use exercise to enhance my social life (for example, exercise with friends)?

_____

_____

Diet

What is my current eating schedule (3 meals a day, snacks, beverages, etc.)?

_____

What foods do I eat most often? _____

_____

Do I overeat? _____

_____

About how many calories do I consume in a day? _____

_____

Am I overweight? _____

_____

How many times per week do I eat out? _____

_____

Figure 3.1 Lifestyle assessment form.

Daily Log

Day	Exercise		
	Form	Time/distance	Comments
Sunday			
Monday			
Tuesday			
Wednesday			
Thursday			
Friday			
Saturday			
Sunday			
Monday			
Tuesday			
Wednesday			
Thursday			
Friday			
Saturday			

Daily Log

Day	Diet		
	Foods (what and how much)	Calories	Comments
Sunday			
Monday			
Tuesday			
Wednesday			
Thursday			
Friday			
Saturday			
Sunday			
Monday			
Tuesday			
Wednesday			
Thursday			
Friday			
Saturday			

thinking about what you know about diabetes. If you have read this far into the book, you have more than enough information on what diabetes is and how it can affect you and how you can affect it. This is a considerable amount of information to know about your disease. You know more about your disease process than many others know about their medical problems. You are up to the personal challenges that lie ahead.

The next question to ask yourself, as the spaceship project planner did, is whether you have the right resources to create a successful action plan. Most of the resources that you need are likely already in place. The mere fact that you have been reading this book shows that you have no difficulty finding resources. I'm sure that you've spoken with someone who has diabetes or that knows about someone who does. That person along with other family and friends will be your support group and will help you plan your new lifestyle. They may even be a significant part of it.

Recognizing Necessary Changes

Nearly all of us understand that change can be good without coming easy. In fact, some of the most difficult changes we make in our lives can be the most rewarding. I'm sure everyone reading this book has at least one story that validates this point. But sometimes recognizing what you need to change in your life to allow you to succeed can be difficult.

Let's look at three principles that you must abide by to help you recognize changes you need to make in your lifestyle.

First, if you have type 2 diabetes, then you must do some form of exercise. I'm certain that you understand this point, and I will not belabor it. But I will cover some helpful ways to incorporate exercise into your life without losing balance.

Second, you must control your food consumption. Easy to do? Absolutely not, but in chapter 5, I'll discuss ways to overcome this often-difficult obstacle.

Third, you must allow yourself to make mistakes. But more important, you must learn from your mistakes. Just as the spaceship project planner performs the thousands of calculations to refine her plan, this is the process that will help you refine your plan for a healthy lifestyle.

To ensure success, your lifestyle plan must incorporate these three principles. (The following chapters discuss these issues in more detail.)

Defining Your Lifestyle

Everyone has different needs and different likes and dislikes. But diabetes can affect everyone in very similar ways, and this is what gives all people with the disease a common thread when developing an action plan for diabetes.

Three Principles of a Healthy Lifestyle

1. I must exercise.
2. I must control food consumption.
3. I must learn from mistakes to improve my action plan for diabetes.

Some of us like to run for exercise, whereas others prefer swimming. These are two very different activities, yet they both can contribute to treating diabetes. The point is that you need to do some form of exercise and, more important, it should be exercise that you enjoy doing and that you can realistically incorporate into your daily life. If you choose an exercise now and it later becomes problematic for you, whether you become bored with it or you are unable to physically do it because of an injury, do not be afraid to change it.

The same principle applies to your eating habits. For example, if you're not a vegetarian and you never found a reason to be, then don't become one. Many people, including myself, who know that they need change in their lives will try to adopt the lifestyle of someone else. At first it seems like a good idea, but when they finally realize that they have their own needs, desires, and tastes that conflict with that person's needs, desires, and tastes, it does not seem like such a wise choice.

When I was a medical student I felt the need to make a change in my lifestyle. I was somewhat overweight and had not done any significant exercise for at least two years. A friend and classmate of mine was a vegetarian and very fit. He would always find time to work out and was very energetic. As most of us would do, I compared myself to him and this motivated me to become healthy. I thought I could emulate what my friend was doing, so I became a vegetarian and started working out. My only problem was that I like to eat meat. So, needless to say, this only lasted a couple of days.

My point is that you cannot substitute someone else's personal choices for your own if those specific choices do not fit your personality and individual situation. If you do this, you will likely fail sooner than later. But you can look at what actions are successful for other people, and adopt the aspects that fit your own personality and incorporate them into your lifestyle. Simply put, you should create a lifestyle that will meet your health goals based on choices that are compatible with you.

Setting Goals

When thinking about setting goals in life, you typically take a look first at what you would like to accomplish in the distant future. Then you look at what you need to do now to reach your ultimate goal. We create the

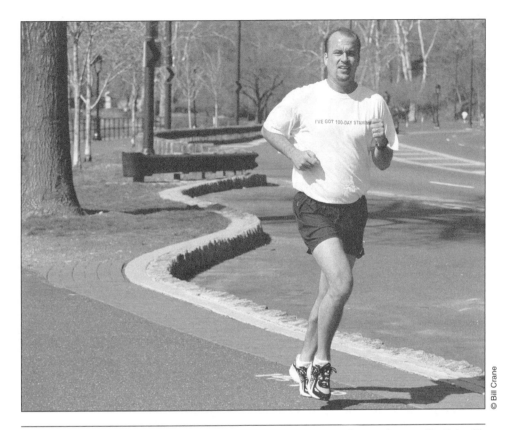

© Bill Crane

Make sure the type of exercise you choose is something you enjoy so that you'll stick with it.

building blocks, or short-term goals, that you can stack together to realize a long-term goal. I recommend doing the same when setting goals for your health.

Take a look at where you are in regard to health status, and then think about where you would ultimately like to be. For example, Kathy, whom we will discuss in chapter 6, is an overweight person who has recently been diagnosed with type 2 diabetes. She is not on a diet or exercise program. Her ultimate goal is to lose weight, become an active person who competes in charity runs, and avoid having to take medication to control her glucose. Obviously, without training for the charity run, she will likely not succeed in the race. So her short-term goal (building block) will be to start an exercise program slowly and safely. As a result of learning how to improve her eating habits, she will start to lose weight. Then when Kathy's fitness level improves she will begin to train for her race. Her goal of not taking medication will be in line with increasing her insulin sensitivity through exercise. She has to realize what her long-term goals are and then set up a plan or a series of short-term goals to achieve these ultimate goals.

You may have a long-term goal similar to Kathy's, and you may have more or less detailed goals. But exercise and diet goals all have similar results—glucose control. Take a moment to consider your three most important long-term goals. Using table 3.2 as an example, write them down on the chart provided in table 3.3. Then think of the short-term goals, starting with an easily attainable goal (level 1) and working your way up to a more specific short-term goal (level 4), which you can add together to achieve your long-term goal.

Changing Your Perspective

How many times have your heard someone say in conversation, "Well, look at it this way . . .," and found that their words gave you a new and sensible perspective on an issue? I have been in many of these situations, and I have been able to come up with many solutions to problems as a result. I would like to offer you a different way to look at how you can go about planning for a healthier lifestyle.

We all know that we have existed in the past, and all that we have done in the past affects us in the present. And the things we do in the present will come to pass and therefore affect our futures. Although this sounds obvious, we often question how things have evolved that have led to our

Table 3.2   Sample Goal-Setting Chart

Long-term goals	Short-term goals, level 1	Short-term goals, level 2	Short-term goals, level 3	Short-term goals, level 4
1. Glucose control	See health care team for recommendations	Measure blood glucose 1 to 2 times per day(for oral hypoglycemic agents)	Decrease calories in daily diet from 1,800 to 1,600	Stick to 1,600-calorie diet Exercise 5 to 7 days per week
2. Lose 10 pounds	See health care team for recommendations	Increase frequency of walking from 4 to 5 days a week	Eat fewer calories (as above)	Stick to 1,600-calorie diet Exercise 5 to 7 days per week
3. Run 5K race	See health care team for recommendations	Substitute jogging or running for walking one day a week	Walk for 20 minutes 4 to 5 times per week	Sign up for the local charity 5K Run 30 minutes 5 to 7 days per week

Table 3.3 Your Goal-Setting Chart

Long-term goals	Short-term goal, level 1	Short term goals, level 2	Short-term goals, level 3	Short-term goals, level 4
1.				
2.				
3.				

current situation, without taking into account our past actions. For instance, we may ask, "How did my health get so out of hand?" Some of my patients gain insight into their own situation by thinking about their lives in this way. I ask them to think of themselves as three different people: their past, present, and future persons.

Your Past Person

It's likely that your past person is directly responsible for your current condition. This past person is not changeable; what that person has done has already taken place, but the results of what that person did may not have fully come to pass. For instance, if you had not been exercising and eating well, then you likely have gained weight and may have a poor lipid profile or other related problems. But as I explain in detail in this book, these situations are changeable. If your current person acts to eliminate the problems caused by past behaviors, your future person will not suffer the consequences.

Your Present Person

This is the person who has created your past and perpetually waits to live your future; it is your master person. Recognize that what you do today will in some form affect your present person tomorrow. So your expectations of your action plan should be based on your present person. Use this book to gain a better understanding of how diabetes has affected your past person and how it will affect your future person if your present person does not change. From this, create your plan to make changes in your current actions and habits, and carry that into your future.

Your Future Person

Your future is really now, and the same will be true tomorrow as well. I am sure that you have heard similar statements, and you may find them cliché. But think about this in this way: We are creatures of time and cannot really experience our "true" future because we will always live our lives in the present. However, we can think of our futures as change in our present lives. Currently you may not be there; you may see changes that need to take place. Use this book to help you make changes now that will positively affect you later.

I hope this way of thinking helps you gain a new perspective on the control you have over your life, as it has for me and some of my patients.

PLANNING YOUR LIFESTYLE

☐ Use the Lifestyle Assessment Form to get an idea of your attitudes toward exercise and eating.

☐ Monitor your exercise and eating habits daily for two weeks and record your findings on the form.

☐ Recognize where you need to change in the areas of exercise and diet, and customize these changes to fit your needs, likes, and dislikes (for example, what exercise do *you* like to do?).

☐ Find or acquire the resources and support group to help you stay informed about diabetes.

☐ Set specific and measurable goals for improving your exercise level and diet.

☐ Gain a new perspective on how change occurs in your life by recognizing your past, present, and future persons.

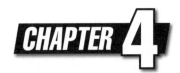
MAKING EXERCISE WORK FOR YOU

U p to this point we have focused on tools for your action plan for diabetes. In this chapter we focus on the main components of your plan: exercise and how it relates to eating and weight control. Chapter 5 goes into more detail about nutrition and weight management.

It is important to note that any change either in exercise habits or in eating habits will directly affect your weight. For instance, if you decrease your physical activity and increase your caloric intake, then you will gain weight. The body stores excess calories mainly as fat. If you increase your physical activity and keep your caloric intake stable or decrease it, you will lose weight. To maintain a stable weight, you simply maintain the energy (calories) you put into your body and maintain the energy you use (exercise). This is called energy balance (see table 4.1). If there is less energy put into a system than the system consumes, then the system will

Table 4.1   Energy Balance Chart

Energy in = food consumption

Energy out = energy used for exercise and normal body functions

Energy balance	Result
Energy in = energy out	Weight stable
Energy in > energy out	Weight gain
Energy in < energy out	Weight loss

operate at a deficit, requiring energy from another source, such as stored fat in the body. On the other hand, if the amount of energy put into the system is greater than the energy consumed, then that system will be operating under an excessive load. The concept is simple, and putting it into action can be, too, if you plan carefully.

What Is the Evidence?

Exercise can enhance glucose metabolism, preventing the onset of type 2 diabetes. One study (Manson et al. 1991) looked at nearly 90,000 middle-aged women over an eight-year period. The results demonstrated that those who exercise vigorously at least one time per week have a lower risk of developing diabetes. The same study also showed that those who exercise and are significantly overweight have a similar benefit. A more recent study (Hu et al. 1999) looked at 70,000 people and found that the exercise does not have to be as vigorous as once thought to have the same preventive effects.

Through many studies we have found that exercise also decreases heart disease risk. One study of women (Lee et al. 2001) demonstrated that light to moderate activity is associated with decreased heart disease. But regardless of sex or health status, most people who exercise will improve their blood pressure and cholesterol, reduce body fat, and reduce glucose levels—that is, they will experience changes that are especially important for those with diabetes. We also have evidence that shows that exercise may decrease symptom anxiety, relieve depression, improve work productivity, and reduce the risks for certain types of cancer.

Preexercise Consultation and Exam

You need to consult your physician before you start an exercise program. If you have type 1 diabetes, your risks associated with exercise are higher than they are for someone with type 2. In addition, those with type 1 diabetes are usually at or below their ideal body weight. So if you have type 1 diabetes, you should look at exercising as a means of improving your overall health rather than losing weight. For example, if you have type 1 diabetes and you have high cholesterol, you can improve your cholesterol with exercise regardless of your body composition (Laaksonen et al. 2000). If you have type 2 diabetes, achieving and maintaining a healthy weight will be most important in thriving with diabetes.

If you've been diagnosed with diabetes but you have not experienced any noticeable symptoms, you should still visit with your physician to review your health risks. Those with diabetes have an average of three times the risk of having high cholesterol and triglycerides than those without diabetes. This is also referred to as dyslipidemia, a condition in which the blood levels of "bad" cholesterol (LDL or low-density lipids) and triglycerides are too high and levels of "good" cholesterol (HDL or high-density lipids) are too low. This diagnosis alone can increase your risk of heart problems and should be addressed by your health care provider.

Unfortunately, many patients diagnosed with diabetes are not counseled on the benefits of exercise. In fact, one study (Wee et al. 1999) published in the *Journal of the American Medical Association* shows that only 34 percent of physicians counsel their patients about exercise. In today's medical environment of managed care, it has become more difficult for physicians to spend time counseling their patients on exercise. Many patients are turning to nurses who specialize in diabetes education, which is important to your overall care.

The American Diabetes Association has developed an easy way to remember three main targets to strive for to prevent complications, mainly heart disease. These targets are known as the ABCs (see table 4.2). The letter A represents A_{1C}, or hemoglobin A_{1C}, which is a measure of your average glucose level over the last three months. The ideal level is less than 7 percent and should be evaluated at least twice per year. The B is for blood pressure, which should be checked at each visit with a physician or nurse, and it should be less than 130/80 mmHg. The letter C is for cholesterol, specifically LDL (bad cholesterol). Your LDL should be monitored at least once a year and ideally will be less than 100 mg/dl.

Table 4.2 The American Diabetes Association ABCs

ADA's ABC	Recommended evaluation (minimal)	Recommended levels
A: A_{1C} (hemoglobin A_{1C})	Twice a year	<7%
B: Blood pressure	Each office visit	<130/80 mmHg
C: Cholesterol (LDL)	Yearly	<100 mg/dl

At your preexercise consultation and exam, your physician will determine whether you have conditions and risks (diabetes-related or not) that can interfere with your exercise program. Certain screenings should be done in those with diabetes and in all people in certain age groups. Besides the main risk of cardiovascular disease, there are other risks that your physician must determine. The following list summarizes these risks so that you can be aware of what to expect during the visit with your doctor.

- **Peripheral Vascular Disease.** The symptoms include pain in the legs while walking (known as intermittent claudication), hair loss, cold feet, decreased pulse rate, and thinning of the tissues in the extremities. By restricting blood flow to the extremities, peripheral vascular disease can hinder proper muscle function. See chapter 2 to review specifics about peripheral vascular disease.

- **Peripheral Neuropathy.** Symptoms include decreased sensation and burning sensation in the extremities, especially the feet. More extreme symptoms such as numbness or pain in the limbs or decreased control of the muscles or the bowels or bladder can also signal problems with peripheral nerve function. See chapter 2 and the section called "Risks of Exercising With Diabetes" in this chapter to review specifics about peripheral neuropathy.

- **Eye Disease.** Visual difficulties of any kind including symptoms such as blurred vision should be taken seriously. As discussed in chapter 2, all people with type 1 diabetes should have annual eye exams, and all people with type 2 diabetes should receive an eye exam by an ophthalmologist at the onset of their diagnosis.

- **Autonomic Neuropathy.** The main symptoms of autonomic neuropathy as it relates to exercise include heat intolerance, the inability to sense hypoglycemia, and difficulty maintaining appropriate heart rate and blood pressure. If you have problems maintaining an appropriate heart rate or blood pressure, which often result in light-headedness or fainting, your doctor will order specific tests to see whether you have this condition. These tests can be as simple as taking your blood pressure in various positions such as lying, sitting, and standing and then comparing the results. Other tests, such as the tilt table test, may be more complicated. This test monitors your heart rate and the heart's electrical activity, blood pressure, and symptoms while you're in various positions on a machine called a tilt table. See chapter 2 for a review of autonomic neuropathy.

- **Other Conditions.** Other conditions that do not directly relate to diabetes but should be addressed at your preexercise exam are asthma (including exercise-induced asthma), anemia (decreased ability to carry oxygen and blood), and heat-related conditions (ranging from milder problems such as heat stress to severe problems such as heat stroke that results from the body's loss of the ability to regulate temperature). You should also discuss with your physician any problems that you have found that affect you when you exercise.

Preexercise Examination Checklist

Ask your doctor whether you have any of these problems:

▷ Peripheral vascular disease

▷ Peripheral neuropathy

▷ Eye disease

▷ Autonomic neuropathy

▷ Other conditions—such as asthma, anemia, heat-related conditions, heart problems, or joint problems

Enhancing Glucose Control Through Exercise

Before we go into more detail about how exercise enhances glucose control, it is important to mention that the Centers for Disease Control and Prevention (CDC) and the American College of Sports Medicine (ACSM) recommend 30 minutes of moderate-intensity exercise on most or all days of the week. You can split up the 30 minutes of exercise into three 10-minute sessions per day and receive similar benefits in controlling glucose.

To better understand the effects of exercise on glucose control, we need to separate this process into two parts: the acute effects of exercise (what happens when you're exercising) and the chronic effects of exercise (what happens over time). The acute effects of exercise are directly related to the increased rate of muscle glucose restoration (how much a muscle feeds itself from glucose in the bloodstream). We call this muscle glycogen repletion (glycogen is the storage form of glucose). When a muscle is exercising, it uses the glucose that is stored within it; when glucose is depleted, the muscle restores this loss by taking glucose out of the blood. This in turn reduces the blood glucose level, enhancing glucose control at the time of exercise. The chronic effects of exercise are related to the increase in metabolically active muscle. More exercise over time produces more active muscles, which in turn use more glucose, keeping the blood level in control. However, if you stop exercising, in as few as two days these effects can be reversed.

Insulin plays a key role in controlling glucose transport into the cells. When you exercise, your cells become more sensitive to insulin and glucose is transported into the cells at a faster rate. This reduces the blood glucose level. The insulin sensitivity and the increased metabolic rate of exercise together help control glucose levels. You will see these improvements in your glucose metabolism typically within one week of starting aerobic activities. Then you can see improvements in the glycosylated hemoglobin, or hemoglobin A_{1C} (which shows the status of your glucose levels over a three-month period). People with type 1 diabetes experience positive effects from exercise similar to those experienced by people with type 2 diabetes. However, in those with type 1 diabetes, the changes are entirely dependent on insulin doses and diets.

Other effects from exercise can help enhance glucose metabolism. For instance, if we looked under the microscope at a muscle that has not been exercising and compared that muscle to one that has been exercising, we see that there is an increase in the number of very small vessels (called capillaries) in the exercising muscle. With an increase in the capillary density, more blood flow to active muscle increases the efficiency of glucose metabolism.

In addition, weight loss is a common result of exercise in a person with type 2 diabetes and not as common in a person with type 1 diabetes. Typically weight loss will improve the overall health of someone with type 2 diabetes and will decrease the need for insulin in those who are dependent on it.

Risks of Exercising With Diabetes

Exercising with diabetes can be safe, but there are significant risks to exercising with diabetes. Following are several common medical problems associated with diabetes and exercise, summarized in table 4.3.

Table 4.3 Exercise Risks for Diabetes

Risk	Description
Hypoglycemia	Low blood glucose; primary problem for those with type 1
Delayed-onset hypoglycemia	May occur up to 30 hours after exercise
Hyperglycemia	High blood glucose; associated with dehydration and diabetic ketoacidosis
Neuropathy	May lead to skin ulcers, foot deformities, or difficulty with control of heart rate and blood pressure
Musculoskeletal injury	Similar to risks in those without diabetes, such as sprain and strains
Cardiovascular events	Increased risk of heart disease

Hypoglycemia

Hypoglycemia occurs when the blood sugar level is too low, and it can cause symptoms such as weakness, dizziness, shaking, sweating, blurred vision, facial tingling, and possibly even loss of consciousness or death. People with type 1 diabetes are at greater risk for hypoglycemia than are those with type 2 diabetes.

Exercise-related hypoglycemia is the primary risk in the active person with diabetes. To understand this better, first let's take a look at what happens to glucose metabolism in the exercising person who does not have diabetes. The blood glucose will be at a normal level before the person starts to exercise; once that person begins exercising, the body increases the availability of blood glucose as it is being used for fuel, keeping it within a normal range. Many mechanisms enable the body to maintain normal glucose levels, but there are two main mechanisms that you should be aware of. The first is the body's sensing mechanism that reduces insulin in the blood and increases glucose availability. The second is the ability of the liver and muscles to produce glucose.

The body's sensing mechanism allows it to monitor glucose levels very carefully. And when the blood glucose reaches lower levels than the body cannot tolerate, it activates certain regulatory hormones that induce the breakdown process of stored glucose and new production of sugar in the liver. However, in a person with type 1 diabetes, the only insulin that can be regulated is that taken by the patient. And the insulin that the person takes, typically in the form of a subcutaneous injection, will continue to be absorbed, which can lead to higher-than-adequate levels of insulin in the blood, increasing the chance of hypoglycemia.

Some with type 1 diabetes may have an impaired glucose regulating system, making it difficult for them to increase their glucose levels by these most critical glucose-regulating mechanisms. Simply put, if a person with type 1 diabetes is exercising, he needs to have enough, but not too much, insulin present in the body and enough glucose in the blood.

One way to reduce the risk of hypoglycemia in those who use insulin is to ensure that the insulin is injected into subcutaneous tissues of the abdomen. Insulin should not be placed in the extremities (the arms or legs). This is the main cause of hypoglycemia in active insulin-dependent diabetes. Not only is insulin less reliable if placed in an extremity, it also is absorbed at a much faster rate during exercise, which leads to increased levels of insulin in the blood. This quickly decreases the blood glucose levels, creating a hypoglycemic state.

Another approach to avoiding hypoglycemia is to make sure that you consult your physician, who will help you adjust your insulin or hypoglycemic agent and your diet before you start an exercise program. This will be an ongoing process, with most of the changes occurring in the first few months. Your physician will look at your current insulin or hypoglycemic agent dose (if you are currently taking the medications) and look at your recorded log of insulin levels over the last few months. In addition, your doctor will likely look at your hemoglobin A_{1C} levels to get an idea of how well your glucose has been controlled. Once your doctor determines that your glucose levels have been adequately controlled, she will likely have you start exercising gradually (such as walking 10 to 20 minutes) monitoring your glucose just before exercise, during exercise, just after exercise, and sometimes hours later. The reason for checking your glucose often is to ensure that your glucose level is maintained during exercise. This is the overall goal of monitoring your glucose when you start an exercise program.

Note that those with type 2 diabetes who are not insulin dependent rarely have encounters with hypoglycemia. When it does occur, it is usually associated with the use of sulfonylureas, a certain type of hypoglycemic agent. Moreover, hypoglycemia is most likely to occur after you exercise in the evening rather than in the morning. This is due to glucose-regulating hormone level variations that occur in response to the time of day, referred to as diurnal variation.

Delayed-Onset Hypoglycemia

Delayed-onset hypoglycemia is a phenomenon that occurs typically between 6 and 15 (some studies even suggest up to 30 hours) after cessation of exercise. You are at the highest risk when you start to increase the intensity or duration of your exercise program. For this reason, it is important that you consult your physician and monitor your glucose levels frequently before making any changes to your exercise regimen.

The delay in the onset of hypoglycemia occurs secondary to increases in glucose uptake by the muscles and liver. These organs replenish their glucose stores, in turn decreasing the sugar levels in the blood. This repletion of glucose stores occurs even hours after exercise. As you can see, if you do not eat properly after exercising (replacing your body's glucose), your liver and muscle will take what you have in your blood and store it, leaving you in a hypoglycemic state several hours after you have completed exercising. The best way to avoid delayed-onset hypoglycemia is to eat regularly and monitor your glucose after exercising. It is paramount that all people with diabetes receive education on proper eating habits. Typically a dietitian is an integral part of your health care team.

Hyperglycemia

Hyperglycemia occurs in those who do not have controlled glucose levels, typically when levels exceed 250 mg/dl. This phenomenon occurs either when insulin is not present (such as in those who are not taking their insulin or in those who do not have an adequate dose) or when there is resistance to insulin, as we discussed in chapter 1. If either or both of these occur, the muscles are unable to fully utilize the glucose present in the blood. Hence, the body perceives that there are low blood glucose levels, and this starts a chain of events to induce production of glucose. This production of sugar occurs mainly in the liver. In addition, the body tries to obtain energy by breaking down body fat. These two processes cause even more elevated levels of glucose and production of harmful fat by-products called ketones. This leads to a drop in the blood's pH level; in other words, the blood becomes more acidic. The combination of these changes can lead to a dangerous and sometimes-fatal condition known as diabetic ketoacidosis, or DKA. This is a serious consequence of not controlling glucose levels. The best way to prevent DKA is to not start exercising until your glucose levels are safe enough for exercise—generally less than 200 mg/dl. Your doctor will advise you on what blood sugar levels are safe for exercise. However, if you have type 1 diabetes and a blood glucose greater than 250 mg/dl and ketones in your urine, or if you have type 2 diabetes and have a blood glucose greater than 300 mg/dl, you should absolutely not do any significant exercise until you consult your doctor.

Neuropathy

In chapter 2 we discussed how nerve damage (diabetic neuropathy) occurs in various organs. People with diabetes can have problems with the nervous system, such as decreased or a tingling sensation in the extremities, especially the feet. Decreased sensation in the feet can lead to further complications that include a loss of one or both feet. The common problem for diabetics with peripheral neuropathy is the development of skin ulcers, which commonly occur on the feet. You should check your feet regularly for any skin breakdown. If you have decreased sensation in your feet, it will be difficult for you to sense when a shoe is too tight or whether you have an object such as a small pebble in your shoe. If you were to walk around with this irritation on your skin, you would not have the normal response of either adjusting or removing your shoe or removing the small pebble. The continued irritation can lead to skin breakdown, which can lead to skin ulcers. Furthermore, ulcers can become infected; this often occurs in diabetics who do not have good glucose control. Inspecting your feet frequently can minimize and prevent foot ulcers. (See chapter 2, Caring for Your Feet.)

The best way to avoid diabetic neuropathy is to establish good control of your glucose. Many studies have shown that those who keep their glucose at or near normal levels have decreased risks for developing a neuropathy.

Musculoskeletal Injury

In most cases, the risk of muscle and bone injury during exercise in a person with diabetes is similar to that of someone without diabetes. However, those who do not have good control of their glucose or who have long-standing diabetes may develop nerve damage that affects the muscles. For example, claw-foot deformity is a condition that is seen in those who lose function of nerves that supply the muscles to the feet. This leads to deformity of the feet, in which the toes are clenched to resemble a claw.

Cardiovascular Events

Heart problems related to exercise in the nondiabetic population are rare. Various studies have shown that only 1 in 18,000 heart attacks occurs in healthy male runners. And it was found that those with higher physical activity levels have even lower rates of cardiovascular events. We must be careful when trying to put a number on the incidence of cardiovascular events related to exercise in the diabetic population. Heart problems such as heart attacks occur in relationship to underlying disease of the cardiovascular system (the heart and blood vessels that supply it). Simply put, the more diseases that are present, the more risks you have for such an event.

We do know that those with type 2 diabetes have nearly a fourfold increase in significant cardiovascular risk factors, such as dyslipidemia and high blood pressure, that lead to heart disease. So, to know your cardiovascular risk for exercise, you must know what your risk factors are and the extent of any underlying heart disease. Your doctor can help you determine your risk.

Your physician may wish to do a special test that can assess the health of your heart. The current guidelines for such testing (the exercise stress test, commonly referred to as the treadmill test) from the ACSM state that if you have diabetes and would like to start an exercise program at a comfortable pace (a gradual start and progression for roughly 60 minutes), you should have an exercise stress test. The guidelines from the American Heart Association are similar. Both guidelines suggest that if you have diabetes and wish to start a vigorous exercise program (one that requires intense exercise that can cause fatigue within 20 minutes), you should in fact have a stress test first. Nonetheless, you should discuss with your health care provider your risk factors as well as possible tests and treatment plans that can prevent or minimize your cardiovascular risks in exercise. It is generally established that all people with diabetes should have an exercise stress test before starting an exercise regimen if (1) they are over 35 years of age, (2) they have had type 1 diabetes for more than 15 years, (3) they have had type 2 diabetes for more than 10 years, or (4) they have diabetes with other cardiovascular risk factors.

Exercise Types

Before creating your exercise program, let's review some fundamentals of exercise. Exercise is typically divided into two categories: aerobic and anaerobic. The word *aerobic* simply means "with oxygen." Aerobic activities last longer than two minutes and use energy sources produced with the aid of oxygen. Some examples of aerobic exercise are cycling, running, and swimming. *Anaerobic* means "without oxygen." Anaerobic activities last less than two minutes and rely on energy that is immediately available and not dependent on oxygen, such as glucose present in the blood. Examples of anaerobic exercises are sprinting and weightlifting.

Aerobic activity over a longer period increases fat metabolism and optimizes the body's use of glucose (Brooks and Mercer 1994). That is, during aerobic training the body switches to using energy derived from fat during low- to moderate-intensity exercise and more effectively utilizes glucose during higher-intensity activities. Anaerobic training such as weightlifting can increase muscle mass, which increases glucose utilization and results in enhanced blood sugar control (Devlin 1992).

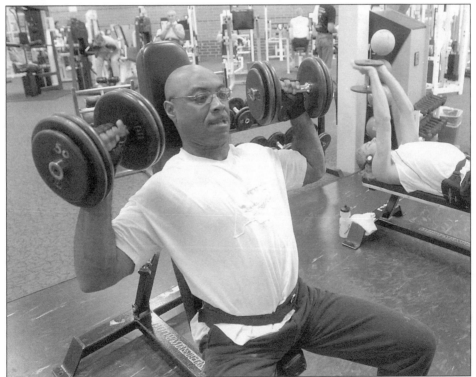

© Human Kinetics

Weight training is one type of exercise that enhances blood sugar control through an increase in glucose utilization.

Components of Exercise

Whether you are creating an exercise program with your health care team or on your own, it's important to understand your response to the exercise you choose, understand your current health status, have a lifestyle that will support your new activities (see chapter 3 Planning Your Lifestyle), know your goals, and be able to adjust to new challenges. It is also important to understand that by exercising you are decreasing your risk factors for chronic diseases, and that the amount of exercise you need to do to is significantly less than what you'd need for attaining a high physical fitness level. Many people starting new programs begin with their goals set too high. As mentioned earlier, 30 minutes of moderate-intensity exercise on most or all days of the week can be effective in controlling glucose, even if you split up the 30 minutes of exercise into three 10-minute sessions per day.

Let's take a look at the five different components of exercise (mode, intensity, duration, frequency, and progression) so that you will better understand how to create a program. These components are summarized in table 4.4.

Table 4.4   Exercise Components

Components of the exercise plan	Description	Example
Mode	Type of exercise	Walking, golfing, swimming
Intensity	Amount of energy used	Low to moderate level: 60 to 90% of maximum heart rate (HRmax)
Duration	Length of exercise session	30- to 60-minute sessions per day
Frequency	How often exercise sessions occur	4 sessions per week
Progression	An increase or change in the mode, intensity, duration, and frequency over a certain period	Increase intensity from 60% to 80% HRmax; duration from 30 to 60 minutes; frequency from 4 to 6 sessions per week

Mode

The mode is one of a grouping of activities ranging from very low-energy work (such as billiards) to very high-energy exercise (such as long-distance running). We use the mode to identify the type of exercise you are doing.

Intensity

The intensity of the exercise will determine the total calories burned, which is directly linked to the duration of the activity. For most people who are not currently exercising or doing very little exercise, I would recommend starting a low- to moderate-intensity and longer-duration exercise program. You measure the intensity of your activity by calculating your maximal heart rate. There are many ways of doing this; the simplest method is to subtract your age from 220. A low- to moderate-intensity exercise would be one ranging from 60 to 90 percent of your maximal heart rate. If you have not been exercising, you should start out at 60 percent of your maximal heart rate or lower and work your way up to a moderate level as tolerated.

To measure your heart rate, feel your pulse at your wrist with the middle finger and ring finger of the opposite hand. Count the number of beats over 10 seconds and multiply that by 6 to calculate the number of beats per minute, which is your resting heart rate.

Calculating Your Target Heart Rate

The following is an example for a 40-year-old (intensity at 60 percent and 90 percent).

▷ 220 − age = maximal heart rate in beats per minute

▷ 220 − 40 = 180 beats per minute

▷ 180 × .6 = 108 beats per minute (intensity at 60 percent)

▷ 180 × .9 = 162 beats per minute (intensity at 90 percent)

▷ Target heart rate (60 percent) = 108 beats per minute

▷ Target heart rate (90 percent) = 162 beats per minute

Any medication that you are taking is an important factor that you need to consider when deciding the intensity of your exercise program. For example, some blood pressure medications such as beta-blockers may decrease your heart rate overall and not allow you to achieve higher percentages of your maximal heart rate. In addition, musculoskeletal injuries may also prevent you from doing activities in the higher-intensity range. If you are taking medication that will not allow you to measure your desired heart rate, then you can use the method of rating of perceived exertion, or RPE (see figure 4.1). You and your physician can decide at which RPE level you should exercise.

Finally, the enjoyability factor of your selected activity must be acceptable to you in order for you to maintain interest in exercise. If you are not having fun, you will not likely stick with the program.

6	No exertion at all
7	
8	Extremely light
9	Very light
10	
11	Light
12	
13	Somewhat hard
14	
15	Hard (heavy)
16	
17	Very hard
18	
19	Extremely hard
20	Maximal exertion

Borg RPE scale
© Gunnar Borg, 1970, 1985, 1994, 1998

Figure 4.1   Borg's rating of perceived exertion scale.

Duration

Your exercise endurance level is dependent on the duration of the activity in which you are participating. The leading authorities recommend doing at least 30 minutes of continuous aerobic activity on most days of the week. Again, start slowly and progress as tolerated. We will look at recommended rates of progression later in this chapter.

Frequency

The frequency of exercise is interdependent on the intensity and the duration of that specific activity. The ACSM recommends exercise on most days of the week for most people. But note that you can still gain health benefits by decreasing the duration of exercise as long as you increase its frequency. For example, if you are planning on exercising five days a week with 40-minute sessions per day, but you are unable to stick to this regimen, you can gain similar health benefits from splitting the exercise up throughout the day (such as 20 minutes in the morning and 20 minutes in the afternoon). The most important factor is doing the exercise.

Progression

Your rate of progression in your exercise program will be highly dependent on your health status, choice of exercise, age, medications, and goals. Divide this component of exercise into three general stages: (1) the initial stage, (2) the improvement stage, and (3) the maintenance stage.

The initial stage involves light muscular activity, low impact, and low level of aerobic activity; it typically will last for four to six weeks. This stage will vary in its intensity based on your fitness level. For instance, if you have been inactive, your exercise sessions may last from 12 to 15 minutes and progress up to 20 minutes over the four- to six-week period. But if you have been somewhat active, you may start at 20-minute sessions and progress up to 30-minute sessions over the four- to six-week time frame. It is also important during this stage to set long-term goals.

The improvement stage lasts up to five months, and you will increase your intensity from low to moderate. Typically you will increase the duration and frequency every two to three weeks until you are at 20 to 60 minutes of continuous exercise three to five times per week. This also will vary depending on your fitness level.

Once you have reached your exercise goal, you enter the maintenance stage. In this stage your goal is to continue your exercise program and reevaluate it to make changes as necessary to maintain your goal.

Calculating Caloric Goals

To achieve your goals of controlling your glucose level, controlling your weight, and improving your overall health, you should calculate the number of calories that you need to burn each week while exercising. You and your physician or dietitian should take into account your individual health status and come up with a caloric goal to meet your needs. Typically this is somewhere between 1,000 and 2,000 kcal (calories) per week.

To determine how much you need to exercise in one week to meet your caloric expenditure goal, you need to know the amount of energy that the exercise you will engage in consumes per unit of time. An easy way to do this is to use metabolic equivalent units known as METs. This unit is a measurement of how much oxygen is consumed per unit of body weight per minute (ml O_2/kg/min), or the energy cost of a specific activity (see table 4.5). For example, if you are interested in walking for exercise, the metabolic equivalent unit of brisk walking is 4 to 6 METs. You take the average of this range (in this case 5 METs) and plug it into the following equation:

$$\text{METs} \times 3.5 \text{ (constant)} \times \text{body weight in kg} \div 200 \text{ (constant)} = \text{kcal/min}$$
$$5 \times 3.5 \times 80 \text{ kg} \div 200 = 7 \text{ kcal/min}$$

When you have calculated how many calories per minute you will burn by walking, you then take your weekly caloric expenditure goal, say 1,500 calories, and divide it by the number you derived in the equation (7 kcal/min) to come up with how many minutes you must exercise per week in order to meet your goal. So in this case we would take 1,500 calories per week and divide it by 7 calories per minute and come up with 214 minutes of exercise

Conversion of Pounds to Kilograms

1 pound = .454 kilogram

Table 4.5 Estimated Metabolic Equivalents for Various Activities

METs	Activity
1.0	Lying or sitting quietly, doing nothing, lying in bed awake, listening to music, watching a movie
2.0	Walking, <2 mph (<3.2 km/hr), level surface
2.5	Stretching, hatha yoga
2.5	Walking, 2 mph (3.2 km/hr), level surface
3.0	Resistance training (free weight, Nautilus, or Universal type), light or moderate effort
3.0	Stationary cycling, 50 watts, very light effort
3.0	Walking, 2.5 mph (4 km/hr)
3.3	Walking, 3 mph (4.8 km/hr), level surface
3.5	Calisthenics, home exercise, light or moderate effort
3.5	Golf, using a power cart
3.5	Rowing machine, 50 watts, light effort
3.5	Stair stepping (with a 4-inch [10-centimeter] step height), 20 steps per minute
3.8	Walking, 3.5 mph (5.6 km/hr), level surface
4.0	Water aerobics, water calisthenics
4.5	Badminton, social singles and doubles
4.5	Golf, walking and carrying clubs
4.8	Stair stepping (with a 4-inch [10-centimeter] step height), 30 steps per minute
4.9	Stair stepping (with an 8-inch [20-centimeter] step height), 20 steps per minute
5.0	Aerobic dance, low impact
5.0	Tennis, doubles
5.0	Walking, 4 mph (6.4 km/hr), level surface
5.5	Stationary cycling, 100 watts, light effort
6.0	Basketball, non-game
6.0	Outdoor cycling, 10 to 11.9 mph (16.1-19.2 km/hr)
6.0	Resistance training (free weight, Nautilus, or Universal type), powerlifting or bodybuilding, vigorous effort
6.3	Stair stepping (with a 12-inch [30-centimeter] step height), 20 steps per minute
6.3	Walking, 4.5 mph (7.2 km/hr), level surface
6.9	Stair stepping (with an 8-inch [20-centimeter] step height), 30 steps per minute
7.0	Aerobic dance, high impact
7.0	Badminton, competitive
7.0	Cross-country skiing, 2.5 mph (4 km/hr), slow or light effort, ski walking

7.0	Rowing machine, 100 watts, moderate effort
7.0	Stationary cycling, 150 watts, moderate effort
7.0	Swimming laps, freestyle, slow, moderate or light effort
8.0	Basketball, game
8.0	Calisthenics (e.g., pushups, sit-ups, pull-ups, jumping jacks), vigorous effort
8.0	Circuit training, including some aerobic stations, with minimal rest
8.0	Cross-country skiing, 4.0 to 4.9 mph (6.4-7.9 km/hr), moderate speed and effort
8.0	Outdoor cycling, 12 to 13.9 mph (19.3-22.4 km/hr)
8.0	Tennis, singles
8.0	Walking, 5 mph (3.2 km/hr)
8.5	Rowing machine, 150 watts, vigorous effort
8.5	Step aerobics (with a 6- to 8-inch [15- to 20-centimeter] step)
9.0	Cross-country skiing, 5 to 7.9 mph (8.1-12.7 km/hr), brisk speed, vigorous effort
9.0	Running, 5.2 mph (3.2 km/hr) (11.5-minute mile)
9.0	Stair stepping (with a 12-inch [30-centimeter] step height), 30 steps per minute
10.0	Outdoor cycling, 14 to 15.9 mph (22.5-25.6 km/hr)
10.0	Running, 6 mph (9.7 km/hr) (10-minute mile)
10.0	Step aerobics (with a 10- to 12-inch [25- to 30-centimeter] step)
10.0	Swimming laps, freestyle, fast, vigorous effort
10.5	Stationary cycling, 200 watts, vigorous effort
11.0	Running, 6.7 mph (10.8 km/hr) (9-minute mile)
11.5	Running, 7 mph (11.3 km/hr) (8.5-minute mile)
12.0	Outdoor cycling, 16 to 19 mph (25.7-30.6 km/hr)
12.0	In-line skating, not coasting
12.0	Rowing machine, 200 watts, very vigorous effort
12.5	Running, 7.5 mph (12.1 km/hr) (8-minute mile)
12.5	Stationary cycling, 250 watts, very vigorous effort
13.5	Running, 8 mph (12.9 km/hr) (7.5-minute mile)
14.0	Cross-country skiing, >8 mph (>12.9 km/hr), racing
14.0	Running, 8.5 mph (13.7 km/hr) (7-minute mile)
15.0	Running, 9 mph (14.5 km/hr) (6-min, 40-sec mile)
16.0	Outdoor cycling, >20 mph (>32.2 km/hr)
16.0	Running, 10 mph (16.1 km/hr) (6-minute mile)
18.0	Running, 10.9 mph (17.5 km/hr) (5.5-minute mile)

needed per week. Then take the number of minutes you need to exercise per week and divide it up into manageable sessions, such as 45-minute walks five times a week (214 minutes ÷ 5 days = 42.8; round up to 45 minutes per day). You should experiment with this equation and come up with ideas for a manageable exercise program that will meet your caloric goals.

Warming Up and Cooling Down

Warming up and cooling down are important parts of exercise. The basic principle is to allow your body to prepare for exercise and to gradually slow down after exercise with smooth transitions. Many physiological changes occur when you begin an individual exercise session that allow your body to function at a sustained high level. These changes can occur quickly if necessary, as when going from a resting state (such as sitting on a park bench) to a very physically active state (such as getting out of the way of a runaway hotdog cart heading toward the bench that you are sitting on). This is called the fight-or-flight response, and it's directly associated with a surge of adrenaline. It makes your heart pound and your breathing quicken. If you do not warm up before you begin exercising,

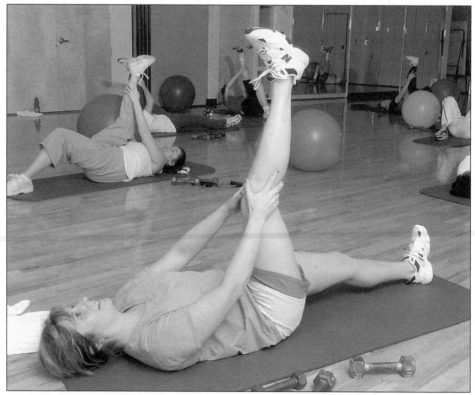

© Human Kinetics

Warm up and cool down with stretching and low-intensity movements—these transitions before and after exercise are important.

your experience will be similar to that in the fight-or-flight response—unpleasant. Warming up allows your body to gradually adjust to the new physiological stress in a more comfortable manner. It stimulates the body gently, gradually increasing the blood flow to your muscles, making it easier to move faster.

Warm-up exercises should consist of stretching and light aerobic activity based on the type of exercise you plan on doing. For example, if you plan on playing competitive racquetball, make sure that you do stretches that focus on the upper body, especially the shoulders, as well as the back and lower body. In addition, you would benefit from light aerobic activity to get your body ready for a smooth transition into high aerobic functioning. In contrast, if you plan on walking for 30 minutes at a low to moderate intensity, then you may choose to do only some light stretching focused on your lower extremities.

The cool-down allows your body to return gradually to its resting state. I have seen the extreme consequences of not cooling down when I provided medical coverage at long endurance events such as marathons. I recall one specific incident in which a man who had just finished a race stopped running immediately after he crossed the finish line and then collapsed. His body was still geared for exercise, and the increased pooling of blood in the lower extremities took blood away from his brain and caused him to collapse. He quickly recovered with minimal medical care.

Cool-down exercises consist mainly of walking and stretching based on the specific activity you just finished doing. For example, if you've just finished running, make a transition into a fast walk and gradually slow down to a comfortable walk over the next five minutes or until you feel comfortable. Then stop and do some lower-body stretches.

Flexibility

Maintaining a range of motion in all joints is important when starting an exercise program. Specifically, tight lower back and posterior thigh muscles often lead to low back pain, which can hamper your program. It's especially important for elderly people to maintain flexibility in the upper and lower trunk, the neck, and the hips.

To maintain flexibility, you can do three types of stretches during warm-up and cool-down sessions. These are static, ballistic, and proprioceptive neuromuscular facilitation (PNF). Static stretching involves slowly placing the muscle in a stretched position to the point of mild discomfort and then holding it for 10 to 30 seconds. This is the most beneficial type of stretching for you to do on your own. Ballistic stretching, on the other hand, consists of bouncing and has fallen out of favor because there is a higher risk of injuring the muscles. PNF stretching is a type of maneuver that involves alternating contraction and relaxation of the muscles; a physical therapist or someone else who is trained in this area can help you with PNF stretching.

You should integrate stretching sessions into your exercise program at least three days a week, and the emphasis should be on the lower back and thigh area (hamstrings and quadriceps muscles). For each stretch, you should reach a position of mild discomfort and hold it for 10 to 30 seconds.

The following are examples of stretching exercises that work the torso and the upper and lower body. Incorporate these into your aerobic exercise program; hold each stretched position for 10 to 30 seconds or use continuous gentle range of motion for 5 to 10 repetitions.

Torso Stretches

These exercises include stretches for the chest wall and spine.

Arching Side Stretch

Start in a standing position with hands on your hips. Put your right hand over your head and do a side bend to the left (figure 4.2). Hold this position for 10 to 30 seconds, feeling the stretch over the right side of your chest wall. Repeat this stretch 3 times on each side.

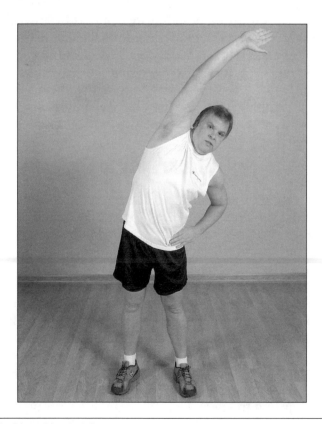

Figure 4.2 Arching side stretch.

Tips for Stretching Safely

▷ Exhale into each stretch.

▷ Relax and breathe normally throughout each stretch.

▷ Do not bounce as you stretch.

▷ Stretch to a position of discomfort, not pain.

Rotating Side Stretch

Sit in a chair. Rotate your upper body to the left, grasping the back of the chair with your right hand (figure 4.3). Hold this position for 10 to 30 seconds, feeling the stretch in your upper, middle, and low back. Repeat this stretch 3 to 5 times on each side.

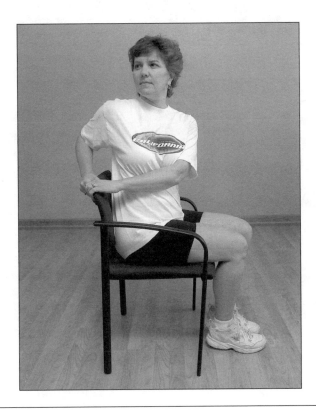

Figure 4.3 Rotating side stretch.

Cat-Camel

Start on hands and knees (crawl position). Carefully arch your back and hold for 3 to 5 seconds (figure 4.4a). Gently sag your back and hold for 3 to 5 seconds (figure 4.4b). Repeat this 5 to 7 times.

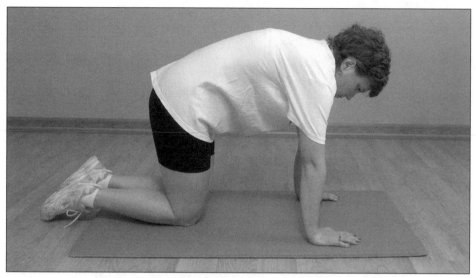

a

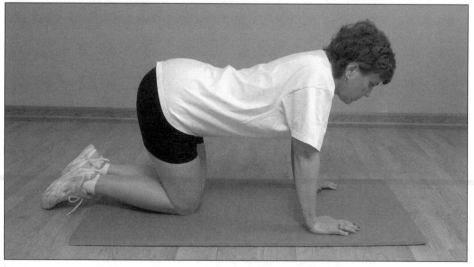

b

Figure 4.4   Cat-camel.

Kneeling Low Back Stretch

Begin in a kneeling position. Sit on your heels and bend forward at your waist with arms stretched overhead next to your ears and hands palm down on the floor (figure 4.5). Hold this position for 10 to 30 seconds, feeling the stretch in your low back. Repeat this stretch 3 to 5 times.

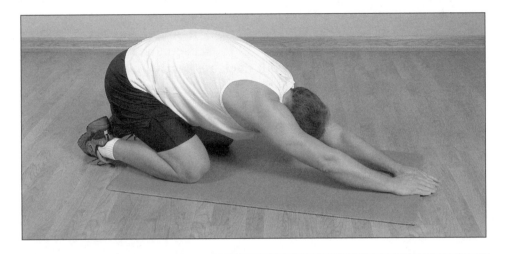

Figure 4.5 Kneeling low back stretch.

Upper-Body Stretches

These exercises stretch the neck, upper back, and shoulders.

Neck Stretch

Begin standing or sitting. Bend your neck forward, bringing your chin toward your chest (figure 4.6a). Extend your neck, bringing your chin toward the ceiling (figure 4.6b). Flex your neck to the side and bring your ear toward your shoulder (right ear to right shoulder and vice versa), as in figure 4.6c. Hold each stretch for 10 to 30 seconds, feeling the stretch in the back, front, and sides of your neck, respectively.

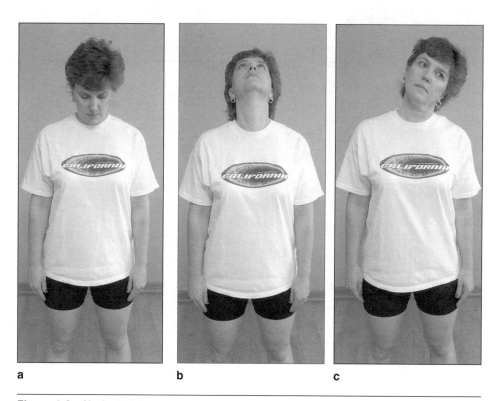

a   b   c

Figure 4.6 Neck stretch.

Neck Roll

Use the same positions as described for the neck stretch, but move through positions in a slow and continuous motion. Repeat 5 to 10 times.

Arm Circles

Stand or sit with your arms out to your sides at 90 degrees. Rotate your arms in a small forward circular motion 5 times. Repeat this in a reverse circular motion 5 times. Repeat the exercise 5 to 10 times.

Shoulder Rolls

Begin sitting or standing with your arms at your sides. Shrug your shoulders up. While your shoulders are in the shrugged position, slowly roll them forward and down. Repeat this 5 to 10 times. Then do shoulder shrugs and rolls backward, and repeat this 5 to 10 times.

Reaching Up and Down

While sitting or standing with your arms at your sides, reach up with one hand toward the ceiling and reach down with the other hand toward the floor (figure 4.7). Hold this stretch for 10 to 30 seconds. Repeat 3 to 5 times. Do the stretch with arms in the opposite positions.

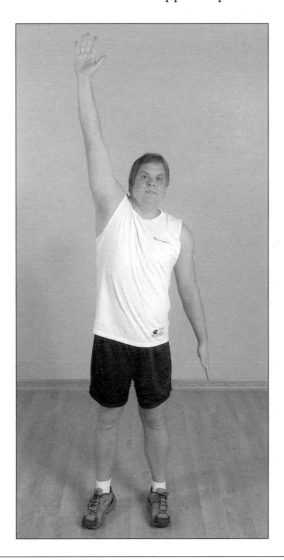

Figure 4.7 Reaching up and down.

Crossover Posterior Shoulder Stretch

Standing in a doorway, place your right hand inside of the door frame with your right arm across your chest. Slowly rotate your upper body to the right, feeling the stretch in your posterior shoulder and upper back. Hold for 10 to 30 seconds, and repeat 3 to 5 times. Do the same stretch on the left side. You can also do this stretch by using your left hand to hold your right arm across your chest, and vice versa.

Anterior Shoulder Stretch

Stand in a doorway with your right arm out to your side at a 90-degree angle and your elbow flexed to 90 degrees. Place your palm, forearm, and elbow on the door frame. Lean forward through the open door, feeling the stretch in your anterior chest and shoulder (figure 4.8). Hold this position for 10 to 30 seconds. Repeat 3 to 5 times. Do the same stretch on the left side.

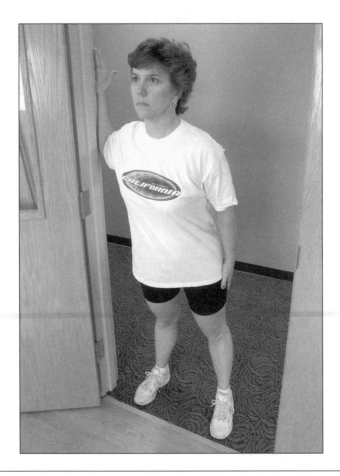

Figure 4.8 Anterior shoulder stretch.

Lower-Body Stretches

These exercises include stretches for the gluteals, hamstrings, quadriceps, and calf muscles.

Gluteal Stretch

Sit in a chair or lie on your back. Flex one knee toward your chest and place your hands around the front of your knee, pulling toward the opposite shoulder and feeling the stretch in your gluteal area (figure 4.9). Hold this position for 10 to 30 seconds and repeat 3 to 5 times. Perform the stretch on the opposite side.

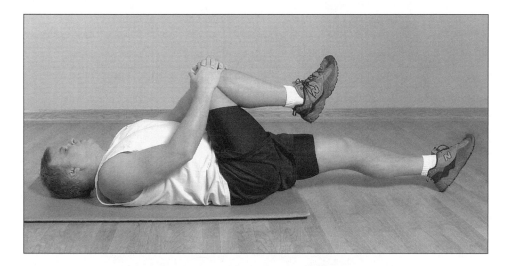

Figure 4.9 Gluteal stretch.

Hip Flexor Stretch

Stand with your hands grasping a chair. With your left foot supporting your body weight and right leg extended back, push your pelvis forward with your torso in the upright position, feeling the stretch in the front of your hip (figure 4.10). Hold this position for 10 to 30 seconds. Repeat 3 to 5 times on each side.

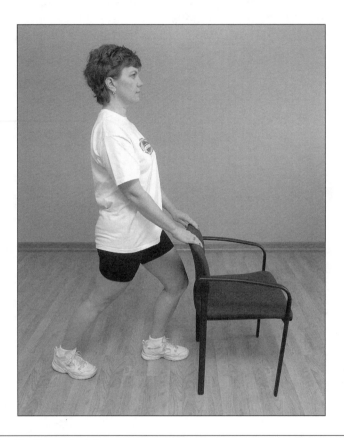

Figure 4.10   Hip flexor stretch.

Hamstring Stretch (Standing)

While standing, place one foot forward on a bench or step with knee slightly bent. While supporting most of your weight on the other foot, lean forward at the waist with arms reaching for your toes, feeling the stretch in the back of your thigh (hamstrings). Hold this position for 10 to 30 seconds and repeat 3 to 5 times. Perform this stretch on the opposite side.

Hamstring Stretch (Lying Down)

Stretching the hamstrings lying down as opposed to standing up helps decrease the chance of exacerbating low back pain or significant knee problems (such as a meniscal tear or advanced arthritis) during the stretch. In a doorway, lie on your back, taking care to support your low back with a pillow or your hand; place one leg through the doorway and the other on the door frame with the knee slightly bent, feeling the stretch in the posterior thigh (figure 4.11). Hold this position for 10 to 30 seconds and repeat 3 to 5 times. Do this stretch on the opposite side.

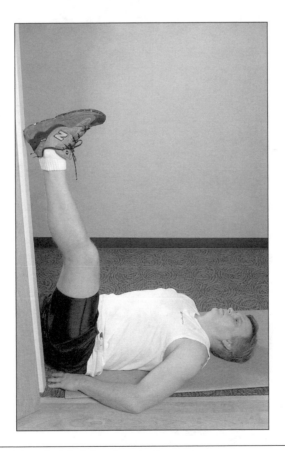

Figure 4.11   Hamstring stretch (lying down).

Quadriceps Stretch

Standing with your right hand grasping a chair for stability, hold your left ankle behind you with your left hand, pulling it upward and backward and feeling the stretch in the front of your thigh (figure 4.12). Hold this position for 10 to 30 seconds and repeat 2 to 5 times. Perform this stretch on the opposite side.

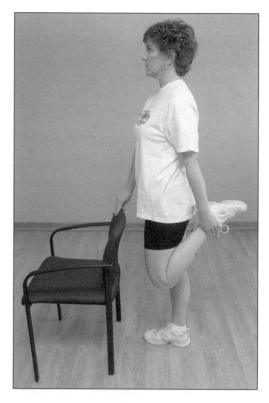

Figure 4.12 Quadriceps stretch.

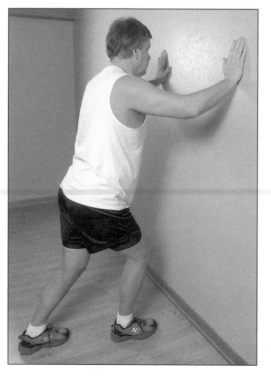

Calf Stretch (Bent Knee)

Standing with your arms stretched in front of you and hands on a wall, support your weight on the right foot with the right knee slightly bent while placing your left foot behind you with the heel on the ground and the knee slightly bent (figure 4.13). Lean forward, feeling the stretch in your calf. Hold for 10 to 30 seconds and repeat 3 to 5 times. Perform this stretch on the opposite side.

Figure 4.13 Calf stretch (bent knee).

Calf Stretch (Straight Knee)

Standing with your arms stretched in front of you and hands on a wall, support your weight on your right foot with knee slightly bent while placing your left foot behind you with the heel on the ground and the knee straight (figure 4.14). Lean forward, feeling the stretch in your calf. Hold for 10 to 30 seconds and repeat 3 to 5 times. Perform this stretch on the opposite side.

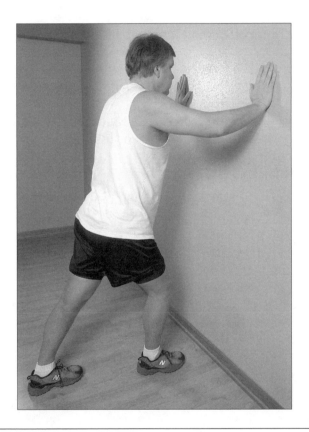

Figure 4.14 Calf stretch (straight knee).

Muscular Strength and Endurance

Improving your muscular strength and endurance helps you maintain or increase bone mass, reduce body fat, reduce blood pressure, improve your lipid profile, and control your blood glucose. Muscular strength training consists of maximum muscle tension with minimal repetitions. When lifting weights or using resistance exercise equipment, you should ensure that the contractions of your muscles are rhythmic. Use slow to moderate speed while moving through the joint's full range of motion. It's also important to breathe normally during these exercises.

Muscular endurance training involves lifting light weights with more repetitions, typically 8 to 12 per exercise. You should do this form of muscle training at least two days a week, and you should do 8 to 10 exercises that work various muscle groups. Follow the same techniques that you use for muscular strength training.

The following are examples of resistance exercises that work the muscles of the torso and upper and lower body.

Torso Resistance Exercises

These exercises strengthen your trunk (spine and abdomen).

Bird Dog

This exercise strengthens the spine, gluteals, hamstrings, and shoulders. Start on your hands and knees. Raise your left arm forward to the horizontal position; at the same time, extend your right leg to the horizontal position (figure 4.15). Hold this position for 10 to 20 seconds and repeat 3 to 5 times. Perform this exercise with the opposite arm and leg.

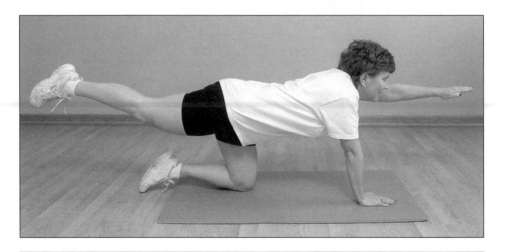

Figure 4.15 Bird dog.

Plinth

This exercise strengthens the spine. Lying on your side, rest on your downside forearm, elbow, and legs. Raise your hips and straighten your body, creating a triangle with your elevated side, shoulder, and the floor (figure 4.16). Hold for 10 to 20 seconds, rest, and then repeat 3 to 5 times. Do the exercise on the opposite side.

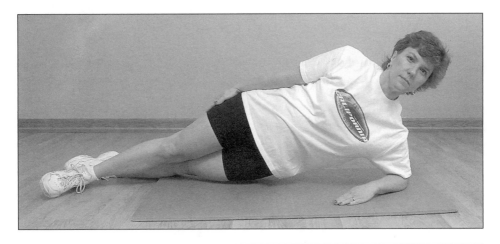

Figure 4.16 Plinth.

Bridge

This exercise strengthens the gluteals and spine. Lie on your back with your knees bent and your feet flat on the floor. Raise your pelvis to straighten your body (figure 4.17). Hold for 10 to 20 seconds, rest, and then repeat 8 to 12 times per set. Complete 3 sets.

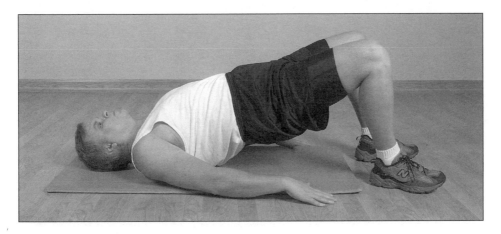

Figure 4.17 Bridge.

Abdominal Crunch

Lie on your back with your knees bent and your feet flat on the floor. With your arms straight and hands reaching for your knees, activate your abdominal muscles until your shoulders lift off the floor (figure 4.18). Return to a resting position briefly, and repeat 8 to 12 times per set. Complete 3 sets.

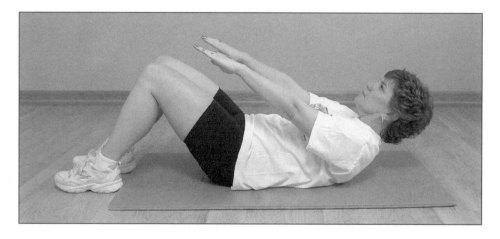

Figure 4.18   Abdominal crunch.

Pelvic Tilt

Lie flat on your back with your knees bent and your hips flexed to 90 degrees. Tighten your lower abdominal muscles as if you were trying to raise your pelvis off the ground, keeping your hips level (figure 4.19). Return to the starting position, and repeat 8 to 12 times per set. Complete 3 sets.

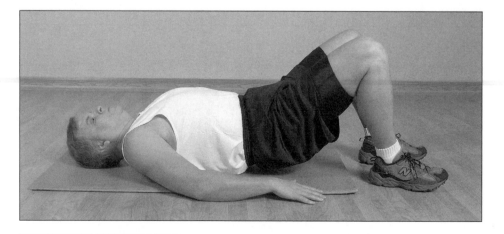

Figure 4.19   Pelvic tilt.

Upper-Body Resistance Exercises

You can use stretch tubing or bands, light free weights, or resistance machines. Start with low resistance and work your way up.

Chest Press

Lie on your back, starting with your hands just above the sides of your chest and holding free weights or using a resistance machine (figure 4.20a). Push the weight straight up until your elbows are nearly fully extended (arms straight but not locked), as in figure 4.20b. Repeat 8 to 12 times per set. Complete 3 sets.

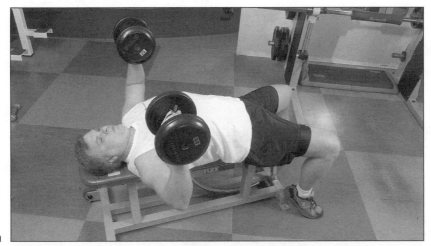

a

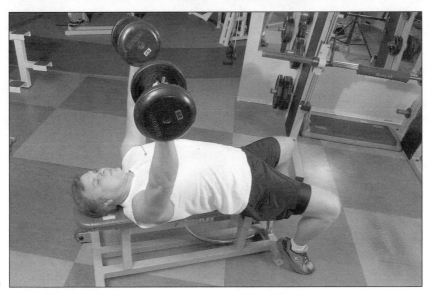

b

Figure 4.20　Chest press.

Triceps Press

Stand with one arm over your head and your elbow bent; hold a free weight (figure 4.21a). Alternatively, you could hold one end of a resistance band with this hand with the other end behind your back in the opposite hand. Straighten your arm by raising your hand overhead (figure 4.21b); return to the starting position. Repeat 8 to 12 times per set and repeat on the other side. Complete 3 sets.

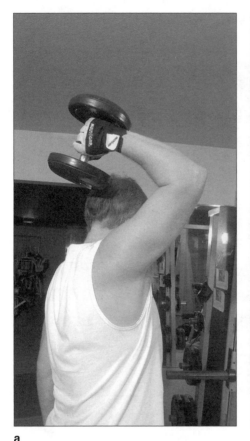
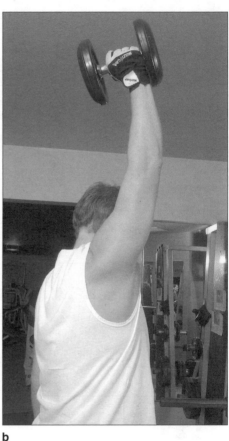

a   b

Figure 4.21   Triceps press.

Biceps Curl

Stand or sit with your arms at your sides and your elbows slightly flexed (figure 4.22a). Palms face forward. Hold a free weight in each hand, or stand on a resistance band and hold each end in a hand. Pull your hands up while bending at the elbows (figure 4.22b); return to the starting position. Repeat 8 to 12 times per set. Complete 3 sets.

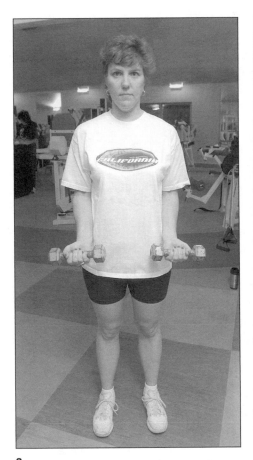 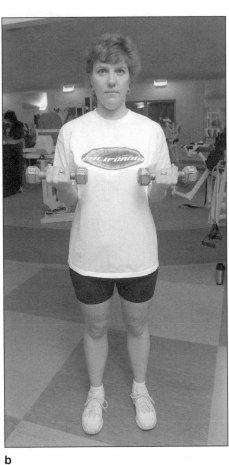

a   b

Figure 4.22 Biceps curl.

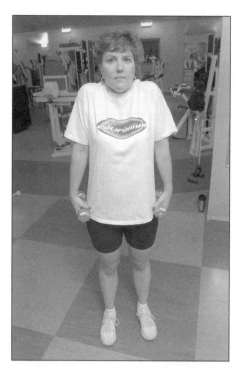

Shoulder Shrug

Stand with your hands at your sides; hold free weights, or hold one end and the middle of a resistance band in each hand while standing on the other end. Shrug your shoulders up (figure 4.23) and return to the starting position. Repeat 8 to 12 times per set. Complete 3 sets.

Figure 4.23 Shoulder shrug.

Seated Row

In the seated position with your back straight, grasp and pull back on rowing machine handles or on the end of a resistance band that is secured in front of you, bending both arms at your elbows and pulling your hands toward your chest (figure 4.24). Return to starting position, and repeat 8 to 12 times per set. Complete 3 sets.

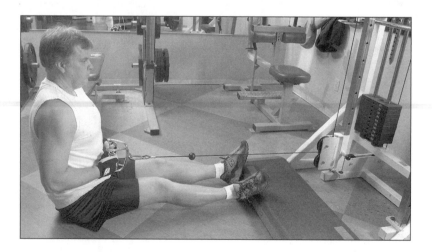

Figure 4.24 Seated row.

Latissimus Pull-Down

Stand or sit at a latissimus pull-down machine with your arms bent at 90-degree angles out to your sides and your hands above your head (figure 4.25a). Pull down on the handles until your hands are at shoulder level (figure 4.25b). Return to starting position, and repeat 8 to 12 times per set. Complete 3 sets.

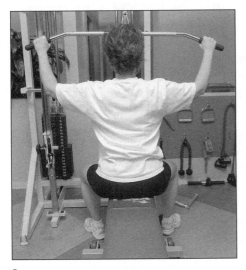
a

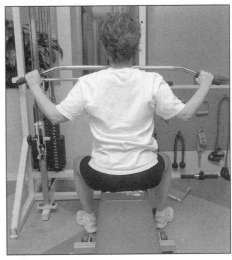
b

Figure 4.25 Latissimus pull-down.

Lower-Body Resistance Exercises

You can use stretch tubing or bands, free weights, or resistance machines for these exercises.

Hip Extension

Lying facedown, extend one leg up, keeping it straight, with your foot coming off of the ground 6 to 8 inches (figure 4.26). Hold for 3 to 5 seconds. Return to the starting position, and repeat 8 to 12 times per set. Complete 3 sets. Repeat on the other side.

This exercise can also be done using stretch tubing or bands by standing facing a table, with one end of a piece of tubing secured to your right ankle and the other end to the table. With your weight on your left foot, extend your right leg behind you.

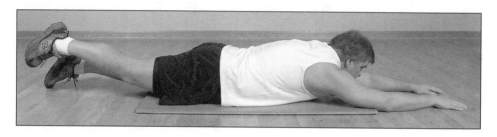

Figure 4.26   Hip extension.

Hip Flexion

Rest on your elbows while lying back. Raise your leg 6 to 8 inches off of the ground (figure 4.27). Hold position for 3 to 5 seconds. Return to the starting position, and repeat 8 to 12 times per set. Complete 3 sets, and repeat on the other side.

This exercise can also be done while standing and using stretch tubing or bands as described in the hip extension exercise, but facing away from the table and extending your right leg in front of you.

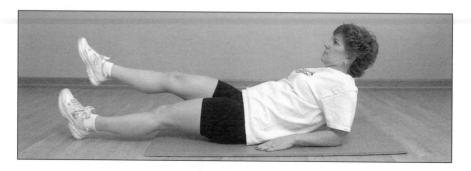

Figure 4.27   Hip flexion.

Hip Abduction

Lying on your side, raise your upper leg, holding this position for 3 to 5 seconds (figure 4.28). Return to the starting position, and repeat 8 to 12 times per set. Complete 3 sets, and repeat on the opposite side.

This exercise can also be done using stretch tubing or bands. Stand sideways next to a table, with the ends of the tubing tied to the table and to the ankle farthest from the table. Move that leg away from your body.

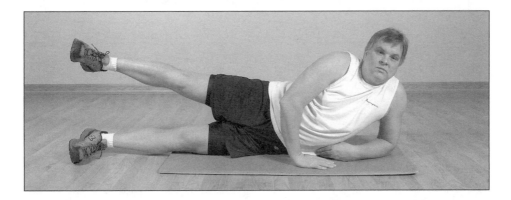

Figure 4.28 Hip abduction.

Hip Adduction

Lying on your side, raise your lower leg 3 to 5 inches off of the ground, holding this position for 3 to 5 seconds per set (figure 4.29). Return to the starting position, and repeat 8 to 12 times per set. Complete 3 sets.

This exercise can be done using stretch tubing or bands. Stand sideways to a table, with the ends of the tubing tied to the table and to the ankle closest to the table. Move that leg away from the table, across your support leg.

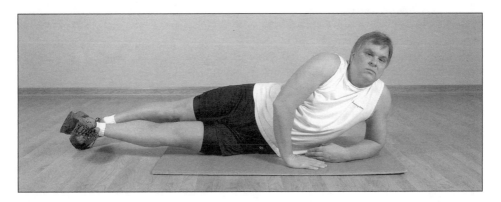

Figure 4.29 Hip adduction.

Internal and External Hip Rotation

In the sitting position using stretch tubing or a band, rotate your leg at the hip against resistance. For internal rotation, secure the ends of the tubing to one leg of the chair and to the opposite ankle, and move that leg away from your body (figure 4.30a). For external rotation, secure the tubing to one leg of the chair and to the ankle closest to it, moving that foot across the other foot (figure 4.30b). Return to the starting position, and repeat 8 to 12 times per set. Complete 3 sets. Repeat on the other side.

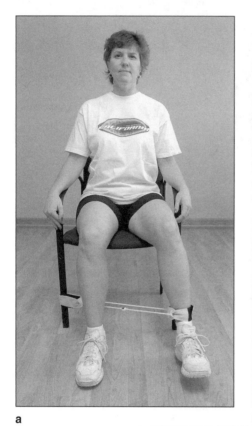
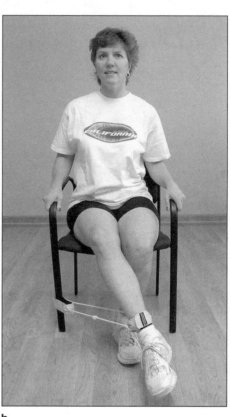

a

b

Figure 4.30 Hip rotation: *(a)* internal and *(b)* external.

Leg Press (Quadriceps)

Standing with free weights or on tubing holding the ends in your hands, bend your knees about 20 to 30 degrees, and then return to the starting position (figure 4.31). Repeat 8 to 12 times per set. Complete 3 sets.

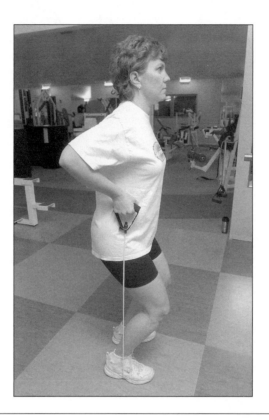

Figure 4.31   Leg press.

Knee Flexion (Hamstrings)

Stand with tubing tied to your right ankle. Stand on the other end of the tubing with your left foot. Bend your right knee against resistance to 90 to 120 degrees. (You can also use an ankle weight while lying on your front and bending your knee to 90 degrees.) Return to the starting position, and repeat 8 to 12 times per set. Complete 3 sets.

MAKING EXERCISE WORK FOR YOU

☐ Consult your doctor before beginning an exercise program. Inquire about the necessity of a treadmill test or stress test.

☐ Understand the risks associated with exercising with diabetes and strategies to avoid them.

☐ Learn about the five components of exercise:

- Mode
- Intensity
- Duration
- Frequency
- Progression

☐ Learn to calculate your target heart rate and caloric goals.

☐ Choose from more than 30 exercises and stretches for strength and flexibility to use when creating your action plan.

CHAPTER 5

EATING WELL AND CONTROLLING YOUR WEIGHT

Now that we have looked at the details of exercising, let's take an in-depth look at some important nutritional information that will contribute to the success of your action plan. Nutrition will be at the heart of your plan, considering that it plays one of the most crucial roles in treating diabetes. Previous chapters discussed how difficult it is to simply exercise and eat less.

We look at nutrition in combination with exercise and how the two directly affect weight control. As discussed earlier, nearly 80 percent of people with type 2 diabetes are obese because of minimal exercise and overeating. Therefore, some sections of this chapter focus on proper eating habits to incorporate into your lifestyle if you have type 2 diabetes. Other sections discuss important nutritional information to help you create a successful action plan for diabetes if you have type 1 diabetes.

Assessing Eating Habits

The easiest way to think about nutrition is to take into consideration the simple fact that we all need to provide our bodies with an adequate energy supply and substances that are crucial to its survival. However, when most health care providers discuss nutrition with their patients, they discuss general eating habits. It's important to ask yourself some simple questions when thinking about your own eating habits:

- Why do I eat?
- What do I eat?
- When do I eat?
- How much do I eat?

If you are able to answer these questions with great detail, then you are way ahead of the game. If you have simple answers to the simple questions, then you are right on track. The most basic answers to the previous four questions are "because I'm hungry," "food," "when I'm hungry," "enough to make me full." But when we really look at these answers, often they do not tell the whole truth about what we actually do in our daily lives. For instance, take the question "when do I eat?" A common answer is "when I'm hungry," which is true. But if we were to ask the question "do I eat when I am not hungry?" the answer for most of us would be yes. And herein lies one of the major problems encountered by those trying to maintain their health through exercise and proper nutrition.

The body is very efficient when it comes to storing up energy for a time when food, the body's main energy source, is not readily available. The food energy that you do not use through maintaining your body and physical activity is converted into stored glucose (glycogen) and fat. An easy way to think about this is to consider when humans relied entirely on hunting and gathering for food. Back then it was very important to be able to store some of the energy that they consumed for a time when they were unable to obtain a meal. But now it is rare, especially in Western civilization, to have a time when food is not readily available. The problem is that our society has changed to the point where food is nearly always ready to consume, but the body's efficient mechanism for storing excess energy has not changed. In fact, most of us do not hunt our food. And the only gathering that we do is typically driving a car to the supermarket to go shopping for food and pulling up to the fast-food window to order a quick meal. Hence, we expend a much lower amount of energy than our very distant ancestors did. In addition, our food now is much higher in calories.

Much of our society needs far less energy than we consume. And thus, obesity is on the rise in this country. In fact, nearly half the American population is considered overweight or obese. And as we now know, there is a very close link between obesity and the development of type 2 diabetes.

So what is the solution to this problem? At this point you probably know that the simple answer is finding the balance between energy consumption (eating) and energy expenditure (exercising). So, to maintain your body weight, the amount of energy that you consume must be equal to that used in the body. If you consume excess energy, you will store it and gain weight. If you consume less energy than you use, the result is weight loss.

This concept of weight loss through decreased food consumption is simple, but to make it work for you, you must understand your individual health situation and set realistic goals. This chapter gives you tools to understand the basics of nutrition and create proper eating habits. However, it is paramount that you schedule a visit with a registered dietitian with skills in nutrition for those with diabetes. Without the aid of your entire health care team, which includes a dietitian, it will be difficult for you to succeed. Your dietitian will help you answer the four previous questions in greater detail. A dietitian will also work with your other health care providers to create the best individualized nutritional plan for your lifestyle. During your visit with a dietitian, she will build a plan for eating well based on your individual goals. She will also take into account any other medical problems that you may have, such as high cholesterol or heart or kidney disease.

Assessing Your Body Composition

Before considering a specific nutritional plan, you should know whether you are overweight and, if so, by how much. This will be a crucial part in goal setting in your plan. There are several methods of measuring your body's composition. Most of these look at your body's fattiness compared to the lean, or nonfat, tissues of your body.

The most common and simple method is the body mass index (BMI). You can calculate your BMI by taking your weight (in kilograms) and dividing it by your

Conversion of Pounds to Kilograms

1 pound = .454 kilogram

Conversion of Inches to Meters

1 inch = .0254 meter

Table 5.1 **Body Mass Index Risk Scale**

Body mass index (BMI)	Grade	Health risk due to weight
20-24.9	–	Very little
25-29.9	1	Low
30-39.9	2	Moderate
40+	3	Severe

height squared (in meters). This gives you a number, or a "score," that relates your body composition to your overall health risk (Mokdad et al. 2003), as shown in table 5.1. If you have a BMI of 20 to 25, this is associated with very little health risk attributed to body composition. If your BMI is higher than 25, then you are considered to have increased risk associated with being overweight, which is divided into three grades. The obesity grading system is as follows: Grade 1 (mild) is 25 to 29.9; grade 2 (moderate) is 30 to 39.9; grade 3 (severe) is 40 and higher. Exercise and diet along with lifestyle changes can be helpful in improving the health of people with obesity, no matter what their grade level may be. But sometimes those with a BMI close to 40 or higher may need to employ other methods such as medications or surgery to help with weight loss. Furthermore, your health care provider may choose to use a more accurate method to measure your body composition, such as skinfold measurements or another tool that uses bioelectrical impedance.

Body Mass Index Equation

$$BMI = weight \div height^2$$
(Use weight in kilograms and height in meters.)

Another important piece of information to understand before developing improved eating habits is the relationship of excess calories to pounds of weight gain. The most simplistic way to look at this is to remember the following relationship: One pound equals 3,500 calories. That is, if you consume an excess of 3,500 calories you'll gain about a pound. For example, if you drank two 12-ounce cans of a sweetened soft drink (150 calories per can) per month in excess of your caloric balance, then you would gain one pound over a one-year period. As you know, the typical consumption of soft drinks is much greater than two cans per month. Many people consume more than 64 ounces of high-calorie beverages more than once per day. They also tend to consume other high-calorie foods, which can lead to weight gain. Another way to look at the relationship between calories and pounds is to think of 3,500 calories as the amount of energy you'd need to burn to lose one pound

Relationship Between Calories and Pounds

1 pound = 3,500 calories

At this point we all know that weight loss in those with type 2 diabetes leads to improved insulin sensitivity, improved glucose control, improved cholesterol, and reduced blood pressure. But how much weight do you need to lose to gain these benefits? The evidence shows that if a person attains long-term weight loss of 5 to 7 percent of his starting weight, then he will realize these benefits. However, multiple studies have shown that, once a person loses that weight, it is important that he maintain the weight loss through proper eating habits and an active lifestyle. Just dieting or just exercising has been associated with long-term failure.

Understanding Healthy Eating Habits

When I speak of proper eating habits I am essentially talking about consuming fewer calories, particularly calories from fat. Fat percentage should be low in the diet for two reasons. First, studies show that, compared to low-fat diets, high-fat diets cause people to eat more calories and eat when they are not really hungry. This can result in overeating, leading to increased body weight and all the complications that go with it. The energy available in 1 gram of fat is 9 calories, whereas 1 gram of protein or carbohydrate has 4 calories. So if you consume a high-fat diet of 1,700 calories compared to a low-fat diet of 1,700 calories, you will eat less food with the same amount of calories because, gram for gram, fat has more calories than protein or carbohydrate. When consuming a high-fat, low-calorie diet instead of a low-fat, low-calorie diet, you will likely feel unsatiated because of the smaller volume of food. This in itself can lead to increased eating, resulting in weight gain. A low-fat diet with the same amount of calories as a high-fat diet will be higher in volume and will be more satisfying and less likely to trigger overeating. The second reason to keep the fat percentage of your diet low is that some types of fat are responsible for increasing cholesterol levels and other substances in the blood that raise the risk of cardiovascular disease and stroke. We discuss the different types of dietary fat and their implications to your health later in this chapter.

Effects of a High-Fat Diet

▷ Eating more calories than you would with a low-fat diet
▷ Eating when you are not hungry
▷ Weight gain
▷ Increased cardiovascular disease risk caused by increased cholesterol levels

Many weight-loss diets are designed to decrease the number of calories you consume and thus result in weight loss. But many of these diets have failure built into them as well. That is, these types of diet plans typically require you to eat significantly lower-calorie foods, often in the form of a meal replacement (such as bars or shakes) that you would normally not consider eating every day. And herein lies the problem. If you deviate from the plan or stop eating these specific meals and resume eating the way you were before, which most people do, you will regain the weight, and often gain even more weight. The same problems are encountered in those who start any diet that they do not plan on sticking with for the rest of their lives. The only exception would be the person who decides to do away with her previous weight-loss or maintenance diet and replace it with one that has the same amount of calories. The rule is that once you have met your weight-loss goals, you must consume only enough calories to maintain your body's normal functioning (including exercise). Otherwise, if you eat more food than you need, you will gain weight.

Pitfalls of Fad Dieting

For many reasons, fad diets are not trustworthy ways to lose weight and also remain healthy. They can also be difficult to stick with. Here are a few of the reasons:

▷ They are usually expensive.

▷ People get bored with the diet-plan foods.

▷ People usually stop the diet plan and regain weight.

▷ The diets are difficult to continue for a lifetime.

▷ The diets typically do not include exercise plans.

Your taste in foods may change, and this is normal, even healthy. However, in light of this fact, you will need guidance from your health care team, particularly your dietitian. A dietitian can help you incorporate changes into your lifestyle as your taste in food changes.

In hopes of avoiding confusion, I make reference to the most recent nutritional principles and recommendations given by the American Diabetes Association, which are commonly referenced by registered dietitians who consult with people who have diabetes. Your dietitian will create a specific diet plan that will incorporate the following basic nutritional principles.

Nutrition Basics

Let's look at each of the basic components of food (carbohydrates, proteins, and fats) and how they relate to the diet of a person with diabetes. See table 5.2 for a recommendation on how much of your diet each of these components should make up.

Carbohydrates

Carbohydrates are commonly referred to as sugar, starch, and fiber. We obtain carbohydrates typically from grains, fruits, vegetables, and dairy products. You may have read or heard that certain types of carbohydrates (glucose, fructose, lactose, sucrose, amylose, or combinations

Table 5.2   Commonly Recommended Daily Nutrient Percentages

Nutrient	Percentage of total calories
Total fat	30%
Saturated fat	7 to 10%
Polyunsaturated fat	Up to 10 %
Monounsaturated fat	Up to 15%
Carbohydrates	at least 55%
Protein	~15%
Cholesterol	<300 mg/day

of sugars with proteins and fats) may individually play a large role in the diets of active people with diabetes. You may have seen some diets that incorporate certain kinds of carbohydrates that have been shown to minimize the glucose level in the blood. These diets are referred to as low glycemic–index diets. However, the evidence suggests that there's no significant benefit to such a diet for people with type 1 diabetes, and the studies of those with type 2 diabetes have not shown any consistent benefits with the low glycemic–index diet. Even though there is some evidence to support that these low glycemic–index diets may have other health benefits, most experts agree that eating a combination of these sugars as they are normally found in most foods is more important than trying to isolate and monitor each one in an effort to improve your health through complex meal plans.

Other diets may focus on replacing carbohydrates with other substances. For instance, it is known that people with type 2 diabetes who are on weight-maintenance diets that replace carbohydrates with monounsaturated fats (such as almond oil, avocado oil, canola oil, olive oil, or peanut oil) reduce the amount of glucose in the blood, thus improving glucose control. However, if you consume a diet high in monounsaturated fats without ensuring that the amount of calories you consume adheres to your balanced diet plan, this increase in fat intake can lead to increased sensations of hunger, resulting in increased caloric intake and weight gain because of the reasons mentioned previously. In some people, it appears that diets high in monounsaturated fat stimulate hunger centers in the brain. Furthermore, diets high in monounsaturated fat have not been shown to decrease fasting plasma glucose levels or HbA_{1C} values, which in this uncontrolled setting can actually be harmful. The point is that the key to success in losing weight and maintaining it does not lie in complex diet plans such as the low glycemic–index diet or carbohydrate-replacement diet, but in plans that you can live with on a daily basis, leading to your long-term success.

Starches

Starches are complex carbohydrates from plant sources. Potatoes and legumes (such as peas and beans) are some examples of starches. Some types of starch, such as those found in pasta, can be digested in the intestine and provide glucose that can be absorbed into the blood. However, there are some starches (such as those found in kidney and black beans, peas, and lentils) that humans are unable to break down into glucose. These are called resistant starches. This type of starch does not increase the blood glucose level. In fact, if you replace digestible starch with resistant starch in a meal, you will have a lower glucose level and a lower insulin level than you'd have if you ate mainly digestible starch (Raben et al. 1994).

Fiber

How do fiber-containing foods such as vegetables, fruits, and whole grains benefit people with diabetes? Some short-term studies show that those with type 1 diabetes may have some benefit in decreasing the amount of insulin needed and may have some improvement in their cholesterol and triglyceride levels. However, for any significant benefits to occur in those with type 2 diabetes, dietary fiber intake needs to be significantly higher (nearly double) than what's required for the general population. The U.S. Surgeon General recommends 20 to 35 grams of fiber per day. To put this amount of fiber into perspective, one serving of a common fiber supplement such as Metamucil contains 3 grams of dietary fiber. Most Americans eat only about 10 grams of dietary fiber a day. So to get enough fiber just to meet the recommended amount, you would have to supplement your diet with at least 7 servings of fiber. In fact, experts question whether it is even realistic to consider eating this amount of fiber without significant side effects, not to mention how bad it must taste. So again, my suggestion is that you meet with your dietitian to find foods that are high in fiber that you can eat and enjoy for a lifetime.

Sweeteners

Foods that contain sucrose can increase your blood glucose level significantly, but calorie for calorie no more so than other starches. Your dietitian and you may choose to substitute sucrose for other carbohydrates in your meal plan. However, it is important that you adjust your insulin dosages or other medications that control your glucose in accordance with any calorie differences that result from the substitution. Again, your dietitian can help you with this adjustment.

It has been suggested that fructose be used in place of sucrose in the diet. However, studies have shown that when fructose is substituted for sucrose, it may increase cholesterol levels. Therefore, it is not recommended that fructose be specifically substituted for sucrose. However, you shouldn't avoid consuming naturally occurring fructose in foods such as fruits and vegetables.

What about artificial sweeteners and non-nutritious sweeteners such as saccharin and aspartame? These are free of calories, and you must take this into account when incorporating these sweeteners into your diet. And the Food and Drug Administration (FDA) has approved the use of these sweeteners for the general population as well as for those with diabetes.

General Carbohydrate Supplementation Recommendations

It is important for all people with type 1 diabetes to have carbohydrates available for consumption during and after exercise. For those who wish not to decrease their insulin dosages before exercise, the recommened intake of simple carbohydrate (sport drinks, juice, nondiet soda, hard candy) for endurance-type exercise (such as running, swimming, and cycling) is 15 to 30 grams every 30 to 60 minutes during prolonged exercise (White and Sherman 1999).

If your preexercise glucose is less than 100 mg/dl, it is recommended that you ingest 10 to 15 grams of additional carbohydrate and wait 5 to 10 minutes before starting activity. If the activity will last less than 30 minutes, then you may not need to supplement with carbohydrate again for that session (Colberg and Swain 2000). You are likely to avoid hypoglycemia if you start replenishing carbohydrates immediately after exercising and continue for several hours.

Protein

Most Americans consume about 15 to 20 percent of their energy as protein. The diabetic population consumes similar amounts of protein. Compared to those without diabetes, type 1 diabetics who are treated with standard insulin therapy typically have increased protein metabolism (breakdown of the body's protein, such as muscle tissue, for energy). Those with type 2 diabetes who have higher glucose levels also have increased protein metabolism (breakdown) compared to those without diabetes. However, most Americans, including those with diabetes, consume at least 50 percent more than the required amount of protein in their diets. Therefore, there is no need to increase the amount of protein in the average person's diet. Your dietitian will ensure that you have at least a minimal amount protein in your diet.

Rumors About Protein

Can eating a diet high in protein (more than 20 percent) cause kidney problems in those with diabetes? There is no scientific evidence to suggest that this is true. There are popular diets that currently incorporate high amounts of protein. Do these diets work? The simple answer is yes, they do cause people to lose weight. But in those with diabetes, the long-term effects and safety of these types of diets are unknown. And if you plan on starting one of these diets, you should make sure that you want to eat this way for the rest of your life (to maintain the weight loss). And just as you would with any diet, you should check with your doctor first.

Does protein have an effect on the amount of glucose that is absorbed into the gastrointestinal tract? Studies have demonstrated that protein has no influence on the rate or the amount of glucose that is absorbed from the gastrointestinal tract into the blood. Therefore, it does not appear that protein affects blood glucose levels directly. However, protein stimulates insulin production with a mechanism and potency similar to that of carbohydrate, and this may play a role in decreasing blood glucose levels in those with type 2 diabetes.

Fat and Cholesterol

Fat and cholesterol limitation should be a primary goal in the diets of all people with diabetes. Specifically, saturated fats should be limited to less than 10 percent of the total calories in the diet because they are the primary cause of increased LDL (harmful) cholesterol in the blood. People with diabetes appear to be more affected by dietary cholesterol than those without diabetes. This means that higher levels of dietary cholesterol will more likely result in higher levels of blood cholesterol. Increased cholesterol levels are associated with increased risk of heart attacks and strokes. It is recommended that the amount of cholesterol in the daily diet be no more than 100 mg/dl.

It is known that a diet low in saturated fats and cholesterol leads to improvements in total cholesterol, a decrease in the harmful type of cholesterol (LDL), and a decrease in triglycerides; it also may improve the beneficial type of cholesterol (HDL) in most people. And we also know that if this type of diet is used in conjunction with exercise, it can significantly increase these benefits. Although there have been no specific studies comparing the effects on those with diabetes and those without the disease, the findings are likely similar. Therefore, the low-fat diet recommendations are the same for those with and without diabetes. In addition, a person can achieve better glucose control by adhering to a reduced-fat diet (Swinburn et al. 2001); this is independent of race, age, gender, BMI, total food intake, and exercise (Marshall et al. 1994).

What about diets that are low in saturated fat and high in carbohydrates? We've seen that glucose, insulin, and triglyceride levels are elevated as a result of such diets. However, it has been shown that in diets in which some of the saturated fats are replaced with monounsaturated fats, the levels of blood glucose, insulin, and triglycerides are improved. But it appears that a diet high in monounsaturated fat stimulates the hunger centers of the brain, resulting in increased consumption of food and weight gain. Therefore, if you replace saturated fats with monounsaturated fats, you should pay close attention to your caloric intake to ensure that you do not gain weight, as I discussed earlier. Again, your dietitian will be able to help you decide what types of food you can use to achieve the right balance of fat, protein, and carbohydrate. The following are other types of fats that you should be aware of.

- Polyunsaturated fats, particularly omega-3 polyunsaturated fat such as that found in fish, seem to lower total cholesterol but not to the same extent as monosaturated fats. Omega-3 fat is found in higher amounts in cold-water fish such as salmon, herring, and tuna. Polyunsaturated fats should be roughly 10 percent of the total caloric intake of fat in your diet. Eating two to three servings of fish per week will provide adequate amounts of omega-3 polyunsaturated fats. Supplements are available as well, but you should discuss this with your dietitian.

- Trans-unsaturated fats, or trans-fatty acids, come from processed vegetable oils commonly found in margarine and fast foods such as french fries. This type of fat has properties similar to saturated fat; that is, it raises LDL cholesterol levels. It also decreases the good cholesterol (HDL). Therefore, you should consume trans-unsaturated fats sparingly. Note that many crackers that are not high in sugar or total calories are high in trans-fatty acids.

- Sterols and stanols, which are substances from plants, are compounds that can be used to restrict the absorption of cholesterol from your gastrointestinal tract into your blood. These work because their structure is very similar to cholesterol and they bind to cholesterol transport on cells in the intestine, but they are not absorbed into the blood. Thus, the more stanols or sterols that bind to the transporters, the less cholesterol will be absorbed into the blood. The recommended amount of stanols is 3.4 grams per day; for sterols, it is 1.3 grams per day. These are typically available in concentrated forms such as spreads, since they are present in such low amounts in normal servings of fruits and vegetables. Benecol margarine contains stanols and Take Control margarine contains sterols; both are approved by the FDA. Salad dressings, nutrition bars, and dietary supplements containing these substances are also available. Before adding sterols and stanols to your diet, discuss them with your health care team.

• Fat substitutes, which the FDA has approved, deserve a brief mention. The goal of using fat substitutes is to decrease the amount of fat in the diet by substituting it with a lower-calorie substance with similar food properties. One such product is Olestra, which is nonfat cooking oil that has been used in popular food products such as potato chips. However, despite FDA approval, this product has been associated with gastrointestinal problems including cramping. At this point it is not known how much of the fat supplement is required to provide beneficial effects of decreased cholesterol levels and weight loss while still allowing the diet to be of significant nutritional value.

Alcohol Use and Diabetes

Many people with diabetes, just like others without the condition, can occasionally consume alcoholic beverages without causing significant harm to their health. However, you need to know the following information about consuming alcohol:

▷ Alcohol has 7 calories per gram.

▷ Do *not* substitute alcoholic calories for food calories in your diet. (The general rule is no more than two drinks in one day.)

▷ Many alcoholic beverages such as mixed drinks have additional sugar in them that can increase your blood glucose.

▷ Choose lighter beverages such as red or dry white wines, light beers, whiskeys, vodka, or gin.

▷ Avoid darker and sweeter beverages; sweet wines, wine coolers, heavy beers (stouts, porters, malts), and liqueurs.

▷ Alcohol can decrease your blood glucose by interacting with enzymes, causing sugar to be taken up by the liver, which can lead to hypoglycemia.

▷ Too much alcohol (intoxication) may interfere with your ability to take care of your diabetes (for example, you may forget to take insulin or forget to eat).

▷ Your lipid profile may be adversely affected by alcohol consumption.

▷ Drink after eating to avoid the potential of hypoglycemia.

Food Portion Sizes and Groups

There are multiple food pyramids that are based on the USDA's Food Guide Pyramid. The USDA's Food Guide Pyramid is designed to help you balance your meals in a healthy manner. The types of food you should eat less of appear at the top of the pyramid, and those you should eat more of are on the bottom (see figure 5.1). Other food pyramids take into account food types based on cultures, vegetarianism, and new dietary philosophies. You can find these on the mayoclinic.com Web site. A good way to look at a food pyramid is to compare it to what is on your plate during a meal. Even though putting smaller portions on your plate can be helpful in preventing overeating, you should make sure that you eat more foods from the bottom of the pyramid (that is, fruits, vegetables, and whole grains) than from the top of the pyramid (such as fats and sweets). The foods from the bottom of the pyramid are less dense in calories and usually contain less fat as well. As you progress up the pyramid, the food becomes denser with calories—not to mention tougher to resist.

The foods toward the top of the pyramid are those that we tend to over-eat, which lead to weight gain, elevated cholesterol, and other diseases. I have found that if I eat more foods from the bottom of the food pyramid early in a meal, I consume fewer foods from the top of the food pyramid. It's more difficult to do this if you eat many meals away from home. A lot of restaurant meals, including fast food, fall short of the recommended amount of fruit and vegetables. One way around this is to eat your servings of fruit at home before you go out to eat, or you can ask for extra vegetables and fruits with your meal.

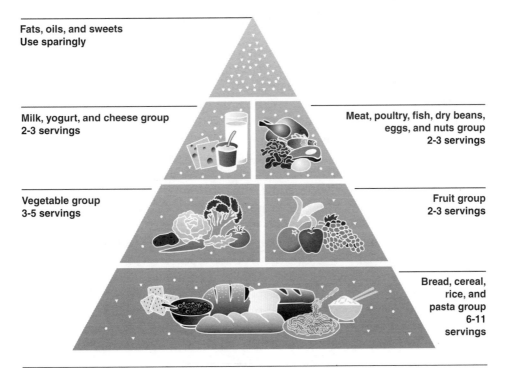

Figure 5.1 USDA Food Guide Pyramid.
Source: U.S. Department of Agriculture/U.S. Department of Health and Human Services.

Buffets

If you eat out at buffets, you will have an easier time getting adequate amounts of cereals, vegetables, and fruits because you are able to serve yourself. However, the problem with buffets is that they are typically loaded with foods from the top of the food pyramid. Eating healthy in a typical American buffet is very difficult because it takes a great deal of discipline. What I have found useful when eating at a buffet is to make sure that at least half (but typically three-quarters) of the food on my plate consists of fruits and vegetables. Eat only one plate of food at a buffet, even though you may think that you did not get your money's worth of food. It will pay off in the end.

You should realize that there are many similarly structured food pyramids that describe the number of servings from each food group. There are various food types to suit ethnic group, culture, religion, region, and many other factors. You can review these pyramids by doing an online search and finding one that fits your lifestyle.

Determining Your Caloric Needs

As you embark on your action plan you will need to know how many calories you should consume through your diet. There are multiple ways to do this, and these are all dependent on your health, weight, activity level, and goals. Your dietitian will be able to provide you with a starting diet plan geared toward your goals. The dietitian will likely have you keep a food log before formulating your plan so that he can see what you have been consuming in the past in relation to your activity level. From this food log, he will calculate the number of calories you should consume in a day depending on your goals, current activity level, medications, lifestyle, and habits. If you are overweight, then you will likely be given a diet plan that gives you a negative energy balance. If you are already doing a considerable amount of exercise, the focus of your plan will likely be reducing the number of calories consumed.

Say that you are currently overweight and consuming 2,000 calories per day. In addition, you have not been exercising and have a stable weight. You have a weight-loss goal of one pound per week (a deficit of 500 calories per day) and plan on doing 20-minute exercise sessions daily (250 calories). You can decrease your current caloric intake by 250 calories instead of 500 calories because you are exercising.

In some cases, such as when it is difficult for you to complete a food diary, the doctor or dietitian may arbitrarily assign a caloric restriction to your diet, which means an optimal amount of calories that you should consume in one day. These caloric restrictions typically are from 1,800 to 2,000 calories for men and from 1,200 to 1,500 calories for women. These are considered moderate caloric restrictions depending on weight. For instance, if you a have a BMI of 28 (overweight) and you are a male, then choosing an 1,800-calorie diet would be a good starting point. However, if you have a BMI of 50 (severely obese) and have been consuming upwards of 4,000 calories per day, an 1,800-calorie diet would be a 2,200-calorie deficit. This would be classified as a very low-calorie diet and would require close medical supervision because of the rapid weight loss and other metabolic changes that would occur.

Planning Your Meals

The American Diabetes Association has created an eating plan, known as the exchange system, that has been proven effective for those with diabetes as well as for those without the condition. This system divides food into six different groups (starches, dairy products, meats, fats, fruits, and vegetables) based on carbohydrate, protein, and fat content. This grouping of foods based on their nutrients, calorie, and carbohydrate content is designed to make choosing foods easier. You can obtain an exchange list from your dietitian or online at www.diabetes.org. This system allows you to keep variety in your diet by exchanging one type of food for another in the same group while maintaining the overall nutritional content of your meals. For example, three meat exchanges (servings) may be two cups of cooked cubed chicken that can be exchanged for another meat or meat substitute, such as four cod fillets. This makes preparing your own recipes easy. Your dietitian will let you know whether you should use this system based on the day-to-day details of your eating habits (when, where, why, and how much you eat) along with your activity level.

No matter what type of meal plan you adopt, you will need to have a good understanding of correct serving sizes. As discussed earlier, many of us have become accustomed to eating very large portions that lead to very high caloric consumption and therefore lead to weight gain. The exchange list takes care of this problem by clearly defining portion sizes. Nutrition facts labels on packaged foods can be helpful as well because they all identify what the serving size is as well as the percentage of nutrients (carbohydrate, protein, and fat) based on a 2,000-calorie diet.

Sample Meal Plans

As I stated earlier, it is important that you meet with your health care team, including a registered dietitian with expertise in diabetes, to develop your personal meal plan. The plans in tables 5.3 through 5.6 are intended only as examples of meal plans based on the exchange system and varying in caloric content. Please note that the number of calories and grams of carbohydrate can vary slightly within each group of an exchange—which can result in a slightly different calculation. This variation is small and has been accounted for in the exchange and will not significantly affect your overall plan. You will need to obtain an exchange list and personalized details from your dietician before creating your meal plan.

General Exchanges:

- One vegetable exchange is 25 calories with 5 grams of carbohydrate.

  1 small (3 oz) baked potato

  1 cup raw vegetables

  1/2 cup boiled vegetables (broccoli, squash, carrots, etc.)

- One low-fat milk exchange is 90 calories.

  1 cup skim or 1% low-fat milk

  3/4 cup low-fat yogurt

- One fruit exchange is 60 calories with 15 grams of carbohydrate.

  1 small banana

  1/2 mango

  1 cup fresh blueberries

  1/2 cup unsweetened orange juice

- One starch exchange is 80 calories with 15 grams of carbohydrate.

  1/2 cup bran flakes cereal

  1 slice regular bread

  2 slices of low-calorie bread

  1/2 bagel

  1/2 English muffin

- One protein exchange is 35 calories with 1 gram of fat (very lean) or 55 calories with 2 to 3 grams of fat (lean*) or 75 calories with 5 grams of fat (medium**)

  1 egg white

  1 oz fresh fish

1 ounce turkey or chicken breast (skinless)

1/2 cup cooked beans (chick peas, black beans, lentils, or kidney beans)

1 oz lean beef sirloin*

1 oz pork tenderloin*

4 ounces of tofu**

- 1 fat exchange: 5 grams of fat is 45 calories with no carbohydrates and no protein.

1 tsp butter or margarine

1 tsp olive oil

1 tablespoon salad dressing

2 tablespoons low-calorie cream cheese

1 slice of bacon

Table 5.3 Sample 1,200-Calorie Meal Plan

Breakfast	Serving size
Mango	1/2 fruit
Oatmeal (in low-fat 1% milk)	3/4 cup
Orange juice	1/2 cup
Coffee	1 cup
Milk (1%, low-fat)	1 oz
Estimated breakfast carbohydrates: 60 grams	Calories: 353
Lunch	**Serving size**
Baked Chicken Sandwich	
Baked chicken (skinless)	2 oz
Bread (whole wheat)	2 medium slices
Lettuce	1-2 leaf(s)
Tomato	2-3 slices
Mayonnaise (low calorie)	1 tsp
Raw carrots	1 cup
Orange	1 medium
Water or calorie-free beverage	1 cup
Estimated lunch carbohydrates: 50 grams	Calories: 360
Dinner	**Serving size**
Grilled chicken breast (skinless)	3 oz
Mashed potatoes	1/2 cup
Steamed vegetables (carrots, asparagus, etc.)	1 cup
Multigrain roll (with margarine or butter)	1 medium (1 tsp)
Cantaloupe (cubed)	2 cups
Water or calorie-free beverage	1 cup
Estimated dinner carbohydrates: 70 grams	Calories: 540
Estimated total carbohydrates: 180 grams	**Calories: 1,253**

Table 5.4   Sample 1,600-Calorie Meal Plan

Breakfast	Serving size
Oatmeal (in low-fat 1% milk)	1 cup
English muffin	1/2
Orange juice	1/2 cup
Coffee	1 cup
Milk (1%, low-fat)	2 oz
Estimated breakfast carbohydrates: 70 grams	Calories: 450
Lunch	**Serving size**
Lean Roast Beef Sandwich	
Lean roast beef	3 oz
Bread (whole wheat)	2 medium slices
Lettuce	1-2 leaf(s)
Tomato	2-3 slices
Mayonnaise (low calorie)	1 tsp
Raw carrots	1 cup
Apple	1 medium
Water or calorie-free beverage	1 cup
Estimated lunch carbohydrates: 50 grams	Calories: 455
Dinner	**Serving size**
Grilled pork tenderloin (lean)	3 oz
Brown rice	1/3 cup
Steamed vegetables (carrots, asparagus, etc.)	1 cup
Salad	
Lettuce	1/2 cup
Tomato	1/2 cup
Cucumber	1/2 cup
Salad dressing	1 T
Multigrain roll (with margarine or butter)	1 medium (1 tsp)
Mixed fresh berries (blueberries and strawberries)	2 cups
Water or calorie-free beverage	1 cup
Estimated dinner carbohydrates: 75 grams	Calories: 625
Estimated total carbohydrates: 195 grams	**Total calories: 1,530**

Table 5.5   Sample 1,800-Calorie Meal Plan

Breakfast	Serving size
Oatmeal (in low-fat 1% milk)	1 cup
Bagel (small)	1/2 (1 oz)
Orange juice	1/2 cup
Coffee	1 cup
Milk (1%, low-fat)	2 oz
Estimated breakfast carbohydrates: 70 grams	Calories: 450
Lunch	**Serving size**
Turkey Sandwich	
Turkey (dark meat/skinless)	3 oz
Bread (whole wheat)	2 medium slices
Lettuce	1-2 leaf(s)
Tomato	2-3 slices
Mayonnaise (low-calorie)	1 tsp
Raw carrots	1 cup
Pear	1 medium
Yogurt, low-fat	3/4 cup
Water or calorie-free beverage	1 cup
Estimated lunch carbohydrates: 65 grams	Calories: 545
Dinner	**Serving size**
Salmon (baked)	3 oz
Coucous	1/3 cup
Steamed vegetables (carrots, asparagus, etc.)	1 cup
Salad	
Lettuce	1/2 cup
Tomato	1/2 cup
Cucumber	1/2 cup
Salad dressing	1 T
Multigrain roll (with margarine or butter)	1 medium (1 tsp)
Mixed fresh berries (blueberries and strawberries)	2 cups
Ice Cream, low-fat	1/2 cup
Water or calorie-free beverage	1 cup
Estimated dinner carbohydrates: 90 grams	Calories: 750
Evening snack	**Serving size**
Popcorn (low-fat)	3 cups
Estimated snack carbohydrates: 15 grams	Calories: 80
Estimated total carbohydrates: 240 grams	**Total calories: 1,825**

Table 5.6   Sample 2,000-Calorie Meal Plan

Breakfast	Serving size
Banana	1 small
Pancakes (1% milk, egg whites)	4 4-inch cakes
Syrup (low-calorie)	1/4 cup
Lean ham	2 oz
Milk (1%, low-fat) or orange juice	1 cup
Coffee	1 cup
Estimated breakfast carbohydrates: 80 grams	Calories: 560
Lunch	**Serving size**
Chicken Sandwich	
Chicken (dark meat)	3 oz
Bread (whole wheat)	2 medium slices
Lettuce	1-2 leaf(s)
Mayonnaise (low-calorie)	1 tsp
Raw carrots and celery	2 cups
Peach	1 medium
Yogurt, low-fat	3/4 cup
Water or calorie-free beverage	1 cup
Estimated lunch carbohydrates: 70 grams	Calories: 570
Dinner	**Serving size**
Pork chops	3 oz
Mashed potatoes	3 oz
Steamed vegetables (carrots, asparagus, etc.)	1 cup
Salad	
Lettuce	1 cup
Tomato	1 cup
Cucumber	1 cup
Salad dressing	1 T
Multigrain roll (with margarine or butter)	1 medium (1 tsp)
Mixed fresh berries (raspberries and strawberries)	2 cups
Ice Cream, low-fat	1/2 cup
Water or calorie-free beverage	1 cup
Estimated dinner carbohydrates: 90 grams	Calories: 775
Evening snack	**Serving size**
Popcorn (low-fat)	3 cups
Estimated snack carbohydrates: 15	Calories: 80
Estimated total carbohydrates: 255 grams	**Total calories: 1,985**

EATING WELL AND CONTROLLING YOUR WEIGHT

- ☐ Review the Lifestyle Assessment Form from chapter 3 and honestly assess your eating habits.
- ☐ Understand the concept of energy balance.
- ☐ Calculate your body mass index and determine how much risk is associated with that number.
- ☐ Have a grasp of the nutrition basics. Know how much of each nutrient your body needs and the sources that are best for obtaining them:
  - Carbohydrates
  - Protein
  - Fat
- ☐ Determine your caloric needs, and then use the sample eating plans to devise your own menus, taking into account calories, amounts of each nutrient, and how much you are exercising.

CHAPTER 6

PUTTING YOUR PLAN TOGETHER

I t is now time to take what you have learned from the previous chapters and put your action plan together. In this chapter I give you sample plans that will help you create your own exercise and diet plans. When you are creating your plan, keep in mind that you need to choose activities and foods that you enjoy and that allow you to be successful in your action plan. Remember to chart your progress, as discussed in chapter 3. Also in this chapter you will learn how to measure or estimate your physical fitness level, which you can use to keep track of your success. Your overall fitness level directly correlates to improved overall health.

Determining Where to Start

After receiving clearance from your doctor to exercise, you need to know your general fitness level so that you can choose activity plans that will work for you. If you have not been exercising regularly, then assume your fitness level is low. In this case you will want to make your transition into exercising as easy as possible by not concerning yourself with estimating your fitness level or measuring your heart rate. But as you reach the point where you are exercising at least 30 minutes a day, I encourage you to use some of the tools described in this chapter to refine your action plan and monitor your success.

As discussed in chapter 4, you will need to choose the mode, intensity, duration, frequency, and progression of your exercise program. This may seem complicated, but recognizing that these elements are essential to any exercise plan will make your endeavor much easier. You may choose to write your plan out formally as I do in the examples in this chapter, or you may decide just to keep track of what type of activity you are doing and how you are responding. The bottom line is to start exercising safely, monitor your progress, and respond appropriately to change.

Once you have chosen the type of exercise that you will do, select the level of intensity based on your estimated baseline fitness level. If you are just starting an exercise program or have been exercising up to a moderate intensity, you can do an in-home test called the three-minute step test (see next page) to estimate how much intensity you are able to endure (endurance level). If you have a low fitness level, choose an exercise with a metabolic equivalent (MET) of less than 6, such as walking. If you are at a moderate or high fitness level, you should select exercises with a MET above 6. (See pages 52-53 for more exercises and their corresponding METs.)

If you think that you already have a high level of fitness, you should have your testing done by a professional trained in fitness testing. In-home testing is less accurate when your fitness level is high. Typically your local fitness center employs a certified athletic trainer who can help you with this kind of testing. These more sophisticated and intensive cardiorespiratory tests and other types of testing (such as strength and flexibility) are beyond the scope of this book, but you can find many references in health and fitness books or on the Internet. Remember that you do not have to test your fitness level to start an aerobic exercise plan. Just start out at a pace that you can easily tolerate. Then work your way up as your fitness level increases, and add in strength and flexibility exercises.

Estimating Your Baseline Fitness Level

If you are currently not physically active, you should start with an exercise program that's of low intensity, duration, and frequency. It should also be progressive, such as walking at a comfortable pace and increasing over time to a brisk walk. That is, the MET level should start around 4 (easy walking) and progress to 6 (brisk walking). If you are in the low-fitness group, we discuss an easy way to start exercising effectively right away. If you and your health care team decide that it is fine for you to do a fitness test at home, you should use the three-minute step test to guide you in determining the intensity of your exercise program and in measuring your progress toward your goals. If your physician orders an exercise stress test, you should ask to receive your fitness level (which is a measure of your oxygen consumption, usually written as $\dot{V}O_2max$).

The in-home test is much less scientific and has not been extensively studied in the diabetic population. Therefore it is less accurate than those fitness tests performed by professionals. Nonetheless, it can be a convenient and useful tool for you to use in your action plan.

When you are just starting to exercise on a regular basis, you can find your ideal intensity by calculating your maximal heart rate (220 minus your age) and then calculating your low-intensity heart rate, which is roughly 60 percent of your maximal heart rate. To find out what your target heart rate is at a certain intensity, follow the procedures described on page 49 of chapter 4.

After warming up, start your chosen exercise at a slow pace. Exercise at a comfortable pace. Remember, if you have not exercised recently, you should start at a low level of intensity (50 to 60 percent). A good rule to follow is to exercise at a level that allows you to have a conversation while working out. At the end of five minutes stop and take your pulse rate as described in chapter 4. If your pulse rate is near your target, then remember how this intensity feels and maintain the pace. If you are below your target rate and feel that you can increase your intensity, do so until you reach your target heart rate.

▷ *Three-Minute Step Test*

This test estimates your cardiorespiratory fitness level. After going through the test, find out where you are on the fitness scale (table 6.1). You can use this test to measure your progress; as your fitness improves your three-minute heart rate will decrease.

EQUIPMENT

You will need a 12-inch step (typical house steps) and a stopwatch or watch with a second hand.

PROCEDURE

1. Start the test by standing on the level floor facing the step. Step up with one foot, followed by the other foot; then step down with the first foot, followed by the other foot. Continue doing this in an "up, up, down, down" fashion for three minutes.
2. When three minutes have passed, stop and take your pulse and compare it to the fitness scale in table 6.1.

Sample Action Plan

The following is an example of a typical action plan that I have developed for patients who have not been doing regular exercise. If you are already doing regular exercise, see the section at the end of this chapter for an example of a more advanced exercise program. However, you can still use the same approach to creating your action plan.

Kathy is a 35-year-old elementary school teacher with recently diagnosed type 2 diabetes but no current symptoms. She has not been

Table 6.1 Three-Minute Step Test Scale

3-Minute Step Test (Men)						
Age	18-25	26-35	36-45	46-55	56-65	65+
Excellent	<79	<81	<83	<87	<86	<88
Good	79-89	81-89	83-96	87-97	86-97	88-96
Above Average	90-99	90-99	97-103	98-105	98-103	97-103
Average	100-105	100-107	104-112	106-116	104-112	104-113
Below Average	106-116	108-117	113-119	117-122	113-120	114-120
Poor	117-128	118-128	120-130	123-132	121-129	121-130
Very Poor	>128	>128	>130	>132	>129	>130
3-Minute Step Test (Women)						
Age	18-25	26-35	36-45	46-55	56-65	65+
Excellent	<85	<88	<90	<94	<95	<90
Good	85-98	88-99	90-102	94-104	95-104	90-102
Above Average	99-108	100-111	103-110	105-115	105-112	103-115
Average	109-117	112-119	111-118	116-120	113-118	116-122
Below Average	118-126	120-126	119-128	121-129	119-128	123-128
Poor	127-140	127-138	129-140	130-135	129-139	129-134
Very Poor	>140	>138	>140	>135	>139	>134

Source: Canadian Public Health Association Project.

physically active since high school and has gained a significant amount of weight. She has tried several different diet plans, none of which she has been able to stick with. Currently she adheres to no specific diet or exercise plan. Kathy has a good base of knowledge of her diabetes and would like to create an action plan to reduce her health risks and become a thriving and energetic person. She would like to remain medication free, if possible. The following is Kathy's medical profile:

Age: 35 years
Smoker: No
Weight: 192 pounds (long-term goal is 152 pounds or less)
Height: 5 feet, 7 inches
BMI: 30 (long-term goal is 24 or less)

Blood pressure: 140/85 mmHg (ideal blood pressure is 130/80 mmHg)

Fasting glucose: 145 mg/dl (ideal level is 110 mg/dl or less)

HbA$_{1C}$: 8.5 (ideal is 7)

Lipids: Total cholesterol is 220 mg/dl (goal is less than 200 mg/dl); LDL is 115 (goal is less than 100 mg/dl); HDL is 40 (goal is more than 55 mg/dl); triglycerides are 220 (goal is less than 150 mg/dl)

Kathy is not a smoker, which puts her at significantly less risk for many other diabetic complications than if she were a smoker. Her BMI indicates that she is obese. Her blood pressure, blood glucose, and HbA$_{1C}$ are all elevated. Her blood lipid profile is also abnormal. Kathy can improve all her health conditions by starting an exercise program and monitoring her food intake. In fact, she has a good chance of normalizing her medical profile without medication, as she desires, if she adopts a lifestyle that includes exercise and proper diet over the long term.

Kathy's dietitian instructed her to eat a low-fat 1,700-calorie diet. She talked with her dietitian about ways to reduce sugar and fat in her home-cooked meals. Kathy enjoys cooking, so she purchased a cookbook with recipes for people with diabetes. (Many cookbooks for those with special dietary restrictions are available in bookstores and on the Internet. If you would like to experiment with your own recipes, a general rule is to reduce the carbohydrate and fat down to around one-third to one-half of the original recommended amount.)

Kathy's Action Plan: Low to Intermediate Fitness Level

Diet Plan

Kathy's current diet is estimated at 2,000 calories per day. After she consulted with her dietitian, her diet was reduced to 1,700 calories. As her BMI decreases and her exercise frequency or intensity increases, her required daily intake of calories will also increase to maintain energy balance.

Exercise Plan

Kathy enjoys walking but would like to start running eventually and possibly compete in a local 5K run. She has not exercised with any consistency for many years and has no other medical problems that would require the need for cardiovascular stress testing before she starts an exercise program.

Mode: Walking

Intensity: 60 to 80 percent of her maximal heart rate (220 − 35 = 185 maximal heart rate; 60 to 80 percent = 111 to 148 beats per minute). She will start at a comfortable pace where she is able to walk and talk with minimal difficulty. (See the section on progression.)

Duration: She will start with 10 minutes per session 2 to 3 times per day (20 to 30 minutes per day). (See the section on progression.)

Frequency: She will start with 1 to 4 days of exercise per week. (See the section on progression.)

Progression: Over the first 4 to 6 weeks, she may start jogging if she feels comfortable, and she will gradually increase her intensity to 80 percent of her maximal heart rate. She can also increase her duration from 30-minute sessions to 60-minute sessions; she may split these up into more convenient sessions as well. She may increase her frequency from 4 to 7 days per week. Kathy will likely meet her goal of running in a 5K race in the first 2 to 3 months.

Resistance exercise: Endurance strength building 3 days per week (two to three sets of 8 to 12 repetitions without significant strain or pain). Kathy will do biceps curls, triceps presses, chest presses, and shoulder shrugs starting at 5 pounds and increasing as tolerated. She'll do leg curls and leg presses starting at 25 pounds and progressing as tolerated. (See chapter 4 for more about resistance exercises.)

Stretching: She'll stretch the large muscle groups (focusing on the quadriceps, hamstrings, and calf muscles) before every aerobic exercising event; she'll hold each stretch position to the point of mild discomfort for 10 to 30 seconds and repeat 3 to 5 times. (See chapter 4 for more about stretching and flexibility.)

Special motivator: The personal goal that will keep Kathy motivated is to compete in a 5K race.

Energy Balance

Kathy will keep a negative energy balance until she reaches her ultimate weight goal of around 152 pounds. Her initial goal will be to decrease her weight by 5 to 7 percent (about 10 pounds) by working up to losing approximately 1 pound per week. As discussed in an earlier chapter, 1 pound is approximately 3,500 calories. So Kathy needs to create a negative energy balance of 3,500. Let's calculate how much exercise she will have to do to create a negative energy balance of 3,500 calories per week, assuming that her 1,700-calorie diet without exercise would put her in a neutral energy balance (keeping her weight stable).

Weekly caloric goal is 3,500 calories per week.

Body weight is 192 pounds (87.1 kilograms).

MET level is 6 (walking).

Calculation: To meet her goal, Kathy will need to burn 9.14 calories per minute to meet her goal; the calculation is $6 \times 3.5 \times 87.1 \div 200 = 9.14$. And 3,500 calories per week divided by 9.14 calories per minute gives her the number of minutes she needs to exercise per week, which is 382. To find out the number of minutes per day, she needs to take the number of days per week that she plans on exercising, which is 4 to 7. So we take 382 minutes per week and divide it by the number of days per week of exercise sessions. To meet her weight-loss goal (negative calorie balance), she will need to work her way up to walking 96 minutes (1 hour, 36 minutes) per day, 4 days a week or 55 minutes per day, 7 days a week. When she reaches the point when she is able to do more intense exercising, such as running, she will have shorter durations of exercise that will help her meet her goal. She will also burn more calories as she starts to do strengthening exercises, which can also be calculated by using the MET units for those types of activities. In addition, she can decrease her caloric intake by 250 calories and cut her exercise in half to achieve the same weight-loss goal. You can experiment with these types of calculations for different types of exercise and caloric intakes.

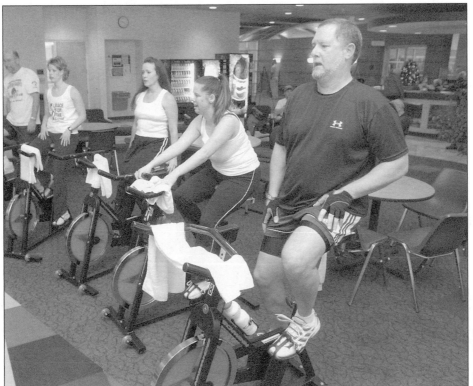

© Human Kinetics

An action plan can include whatever type of exercise you enjoy or have available. Many options exist, such as cycling classes at a local fitness facility.

Remember that you do not have to do as much exercise as shown in Kathy's plan to see a positive change in your health. Also recognize that as her exercise level increases, she will have to increase her caloric intake for her weight-loss rate to remain stable. If she did not increase her food intake, her weight-loss rate would increase, and vice versa in accordance with the principle of energy balance. Finding this balance is the challenge here. This is where keeping your action plan log book up to date can be helpful to you. Charting your meals, your exercise, and your response (weight and glucose level changes) will allow you to see positive and negative trends in your plan.

Advanced Exercise Plans for Walking, Jogging, Biking, and Swimming

You can stick to one type of exercise, or you can mix up exercises during the week. I have found that mixing up the exercises makes my weeks more interesting. For instance, say you choose to jog for your aerobic exercise, and once you think you are in pretty good shape (that is, exercising at 75 to 80 percent of your maximal heart rate), try using one of the other types of exercises in place of jogging. You may even wish to use three different types of exercise. I have found swimming, biking, and jogging to be fun.

Walking

Frequency: 5 to 7 days per week.

Duration: 30 to 50 minutes per day.

Intensity: 75 to 80 percent of your maximal heart rate.

Progression: See the following table.

	Week 1	Week 2	Week 3	Week 4
	Frequency: 5 days **Intensity: 75%**	**Frequency: 5 days** **Intensity: 75%**	**Frequency: 6 days** **Intensity: 80%**	**Frequency: 7 days** **Intensity: 80%**
Mon	30 minutes	35 minutes	40 minutes	45 minutes
Tues	35 minutes	40 minutes	45 minutes	45 minutes
Wed	40 minutes, easy*	45 minutes, easy	50 minutes, easy	50 minutes, easy
Thurs	30 minutes, HW**	40 minutes, HW	45 minutes, HW	40 minutes, HW
Fri	Rest day	Rest day	Rest day	35 minutes
Sat	40 minutes	45 minutes	50 minutes	45 minutes, HW
Sun	Rest day	Rest day	50 minutes	50 minutes

*Decrease intensity by 10 percent, to 65 to 70 percent of maximal heart rate.

**Use hand weights (1 to 2.5 pounds).

Jogging

Frequency: 5 to 7 days per week.

Duration: 20 to 50 minutes per day.

Intensity: 65 to 85 percent of your maximal heart rate.

Progression: See the following table.

	Week 1 Frequency: 5 days Intensity: 65%	Week 2 Frequency: 5 days Intensity: 75%	Week 3 Frequency: 6 days Intensity: 80%	Week 4 Frequency: 7 days Intensity: 80%
Mon	20 minutes	30 minutes	45 minutes	50 minutes
Tues	30 minutes, walk*	40 minutes, walk	30 minutes	45 minutes
Wed	30 minutes, easy**	45 minutes, easy	50 minutes, easy	50 minutes, easy
Thurs	40 minutes, walk	40 minutes, walk	40 minutes	50 minutes
Fri	Rest day	Rest day	Rest day	40 minutes, easy
Sat	40 minutes	45 minutes	45 minutes	50 minutes
Sun	Rest day	Rest day	50 minutes, easy	50 minutes, easy

*Walk at about 65 to 75 percent of your maximal heart rate.

**Decrease intensity by 10 percent.

Swimming

Frequency: 3 to 5 days per week.

Duration: 30 to 60 minutes per day of continuous swimming if you are currently a swimmer, or you can break it up into intervals that you can do easily and work your way up until you can complete the session continuously.

Intensity: 60 to 80 percent of your maximal heart rate. Note that your heart rate will be lower than normal when swimming. With swimming, it has been suggested that you subtract 13 beats per minute from your estimated maximal heart rate before calculating your training heart rate (McArdle et al. 2000).

Progression: See the following table.

	Week 1	Week 2	Week 3	Week 4
	Frequency: 3 days Intensity: 60-70%	Frequency: 4 days Intensity: 60-70%	Frequency: 5 days Intensity: 70-80%	Frequency: 5 days Intensity: 80%
Mon	30 minutes	30 minutes	40 minutes	50 minutes, KB**
Tues	Rest day	40 minutes, KB	45 minutes, KB	50 minutes
Wed	40 minutes, easy*	Rest day	50 minutes, easy	Rest day
Thurs	Rest day	40 minutes	Rest day	40 minutes, KB
Fri	30 minutes, KB	Rest day	50 minutes, KB	Rest day
Sat	Rest day	45 minutes, easy	Rest day	50 minutes, hard***
Sun	Rest day	Rest day	50 minutes, easy	Rest day

*Decrease intensity by 50 percent.

**Use a kickboard for part of the session.

***Increase intensity by 5 to 10 percent.

Biking

Frequency: 5 to 7 days per week.

Duration: 30 to 60 minutes per day.

Intensity: 60 to 80 percent of your maximal heart rate.

Progression: See the following table.

	Week 1 Frequency: 5 days Intensity: 60%	Week 2 Frequency: 5 days Intensity: 70%	Week 3 Frequency: 6 days Intensity: 80%	Week 4 Frequency: 7 days Intensity: 80%
Mon	30 minutes	30 minutes	45 minutes	50 minutes
Tues	30 minutes	40 minutes	30 minutes	45 minutes
Wed	30 minutes, easy*	45 minutes, easy	50 minutes, easy	50 minutes, easy
Thurs	40 minutes	40 minutes, hard**	45 minutes, hard	50 minutes, hard
Fri	Rest day	Rest day	Rest day	40 minutes, easy
Sat	40 minutes	45 minutes	45 minutes	50 minutes
Sun	Rest day	Rest day	50 minutes, easy	50 minutes, easy

*Decrease intensity by 10 percent.

**Increase intensity by 10 percent.

ACTION PLAN:
PUTTING YOUR PLAN TOGETHER

- ☐ Determine your baseline fitness level either through a stress test from your doctor or an in-home test called the three-minute step test.
- ☐ Find your ideal intensity by calculating your maximal heart rate, and then calculating your low-intensity heart rate.
- ☐ Explore all exercise options in your area, including walking, running, cycling, and swimming, as well as group classes and membership at local fitness facilities.
- ☐ Use Kathy's sample action plan as a guide to customizing your own program. You'll have to adjust the specific elements based on your own preferences, needs, and levels.

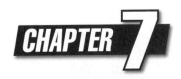

CHAPTER 7

MONITORING YOUR PROGRESS AND RESPONDING TO CHANGE

In this chapter I discuss how to monitor your progress after you have put your action plan for diabetes into motion. As you monitor your progress, you will need to document the changes in your health status in a personalized health diary. This diary should include information such as the dates and times of blood glucose levels associated with exercise and diet. You should also include your heart rate, blood pressure, weight or body mass index (BMI), any symptoms and laboratory values such as your hemoglobin A_{1C} levels and lipid levels, and any other tests that you have undergone. I have found that some of my patients who keep health diaries like to bring them to their appointments to show me the patterns in their health and to record their laboratory test results.

As discussed in previous chapters, it is important for you to recognize the differences between type 1 diabetes and type 2 diabetes and to make regular exercise a part of your lifestyle. People with both types of diabetes benefit from exercise. The main concern for those with both types of diabetes is to monitor blood glucose levels. Those with type 1 diabetes need to monitor glucose closely when exercising, especially when starting an exercise program. Hypoglycemia, or low blood sugar, is the prime risk associated with exercise for those with type 1 diabetes. Hyperglycemia during exercise is also a serious concern in those with type 1 diabetes. People with type 2 diabetes have a very low risk of hypoglycemia unless they are taking sulfonylureas or other medications that are associated with causing hypoglycemia. Those with type 2 diabetes need to ensure that their glucose is not too high when starting their exercise program, and they need to monitor their glucose level to gauge the effectiveness of their diet and exercise. If you do not have a clear understanding of this, review chapter 4.

As you progress through your plan and become more active, you may choose to keep track of how your fitness level improves. Your health care team will track your cholesterol and blood pressure periodically. If you are using exercise and diet alone to optimize your cholesterol levels, it is generally recommended that these levels be tested every six months. If you use medication to control your cholesterol levels, your physician may choose to test your lipid levels more frequently. Your blood pressure can be tested at each visit, and you can check your own blood pressure at home twice a week by using a calibrated blood pressure cuff and meter. You can purchase a blood pressure cuff and meter at your local drug store or online. You will pay $15 to $100 for a simple cuff and meter; accuracy and durability typically increase with the cost of the unit. For $50 to $600, you can get other, more sophisticated automatic digital models that measure your heart rate and are more clinically accurate. (To determine the accuracy of your home blood pressure monitor, take your blood pressure cuff to your doctor's appointment and compare readings from the doctor's meter and your meter.) The key is to measure blood pressure at the same time each day after you have been sitting for at least five minutes. You should document these levels in your health diary so that you can determine your progress in your action plan. See table 7.1 for an example of a filled-in six-month health diary, and table 7.2 for a blank health diary you can use.

Table 7.1   Sample Six-Month Health Diary

Date	11/12/03	12/17/03	1/14/04	2/11/04	3/17/04	4/21/04	5/19/04
Blood glucose	165 mg/dl	130 mg/dl	113 mg/dl	104 mg/dl	110 mg/dl	106 mg/dl	108 mg/dl
Resting heart rate	84	78	78	66	66	60	60
Blood pressure	145/85	135/85	125/80	120/75	120/80	120/75	120/70
BMI	31	30	29	28	28	27	27
HbA_{1c}	8.5	–	–	7.5	–	–	6.8
Lipids (total/ LDL/HDL/ triglycerides)	177/ 83/31/ 325	–	–	–	–	–	130/ 80/45/ 150

Table 7.2 Your Six-Month Health Diary

Date							
Blood glucose (also keep in a daily diary)							
Resting heart rate							
Blood pressure							
BMI							
HbA$_{1C}$							
Lipids (total/ LDL/HDL/ triglycerides)							

If you have type 2 diabetes, a diary can help you keep track of how your lifestyle affects your glucose control. A complete diary that includes your weight or BMI, descriptions of meals, exercise intensities and durations, glucose levels, and other laboratory values can function as an efficient gauge to tell how well you are doing with your action plan. You can also use a diary as a motivation tool, especially once you see the effects of your action plan on your condition. For example, Tom, a gentleman of about 55 years old whom I help with his medical care, has found his health diary to be very motivational. In addition to type 2 diabetes, Tom has multiple sclerosis (MS), a disease that results in easy fatigability and other symptoms that can make exercising difficult. When I first met Tom, he was skeptical about creating a diet and exercise plan because of the complications of MS. He had tried exercising before but found that he overheated and fatigued easily. He'd met with a dietitian in the past but had not seen significant positive results. After discussing with me the basics of diabetes and the differences between exercising to improve health and exercising to significantly increasing fitness level, he felt more at ease about creating an action plan. Once he realized that I was not going to ask him to do what he already knew he couldn't do, we started him on his plan. His plan included riding his bike for 10 to 15 minutes (this varied depending on how he felt on any particular day) and walking in the mall for 10 to 20 minutes on other days. He knew that he could not do these things for too long if he started to notice problems such as overheating. And we designed his action plan around this concern, allowing for daily flexibility. About six weeks after starting his program, he returned to my

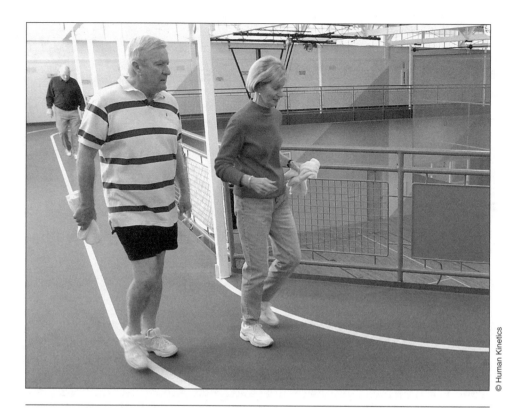

Keeping track of the exercise you do and comparing it with the results of your glucose tests will help you determine what is working and what isn't.

office, and we reviewed his diary. As I expected, he had some exercise sessions lasting 20 minutes, some that were split into smaller, more tolerable sessions, and no sessions on some days. But Tom met his minimum weekly goal of exercise. We made some adjustments to his plan, and then I saw him about two months later after doing some scheduled laboratory tests. He was very excited to find that he'd normalized his fasting blood glucose and lowered his HbA_{1c} from 8.5 to 7.5. From the expression on his face I could see that he was no longer skeptical about his action plan. Three months later, he had mastered his action plan and normalized his HbA_{1c}, LDL, and HDL; significantly decreased his triglycerides; and lost 8 pounds. I met with Tom not long ago and he has had to make adjustments to his schedule because of work issues, but he's confident that he can adjust without a glitch.

Monitoring Your Glucose

Before beginning any type of exercise program, you should be well acquainted with the glucose meter you and your health care team have chosen to use. You also need to maintain the quality of your testing unit.

Accuracy in glucose monitoring is important when gauging the effectiveness of exercise on your health. The best way to ensure this is to have a member of your health care team, typically the diabetes nurse educator, teach or review the proper techniques for testing your blood and maintaining your glucose meter. Most blood sugar monitors work the same way: After you insert a plastic strip or disk into the glucose meter, you obtain a small drop of blood by pricking your finger, palm, or arm with a spring-loaded pen that contains a lancet. Then you put the drop of blood on the plastic strip or disk, and in less than a minute the glucose meter gives you a digital reading of your blood glucose level.

Noninvasive Blood Glucose Monitors

The FDA has recently approved the use of noninvasive blood glucose monitors. One of these devices, which looks like a wristwatch, checks blood glucose levels without puncturing the skin for a blood sample. It can provide six measurements per hour for 13 hours. However, this device is not meant to replace traditional glucose testing; it's used to obtain additional glucose readings between traditional blood tests. The monitor requires daily calibration with the use of standard finger-stick glucose measurements.

The following are some other methods of glucose monitoring that are currently being tested:

- Shining a beam of light on the skin or through body tissues
- Measuring the energy waves (infrared radiation) emitted by the body
- Applying radio waves to the fingertips
- Using ultrasound
- Checking the thickness (also called viscosity) of fluids in tissue underneath the skin

Choosing a Glucose Meter

Many varieties of blood glucose meters are available, each with various features that can make testing your blood sugar fairly easy. You can ask your doctor or diabetes nurse educator to help you determine the best monitor for you. You can also do an Internet search on blood glucose monitors to find unbiased consumer ratings on various models. These ratings are based on ease of use, amount of blood required for testing, cost, speed of results, and variety of features.

Most electronic glucose meters automatically log blood glucose levels; some store as few as 40 readings, and others can store over 3,000 readings. Most monitors are equipped with computer interface ports that allow users to upload blood sugar readings, as well as the date and time of each reading, into a personal computer with the use of special software. Many physicians use this software in their offices, enabling patients to forgo paper-and-pen methods of record keeping of blood glucose levels. Some more sophisticated glucose meters allow you to record your activity levels, dosages of insulin, food intake, and any other data that you and your physician may think are important in monitoring your health. Meters with these electronic record-keeping features are convenient for those who travel frequently and don't want to pack log books into their luggage.

If you have Medicare insurance coverage, you can get 100 percent reimbursement for blood glucose monitors and test strips, and it doesn't matter which meter you choose, be it a simple, inexpensive device or a more expensive, more sophisticated model. If you have HMO coverage or private insurance coverage, you may be able to get your blood glucose monitor at no cost, but often there's a copayment or deductible charge for test strips. Insurance companies offer reimbursement or low costs for blood glucose monitors because monitors are a reliable preventive measure against long-term complications. Patients who regularly use blood glucose monitors end up saving insurance companies money in the long run because patients can control their health and avoid emergency room visits, hospitalizations, and other drug expenses simply by controlling their blood sugar levels.

Whatever form of documentation you choose to use (pen and paper or your monitor's memory features), this documentation allows you and your health care team to spot patterns and make correlations between your diet and exercise plans. For instance, if you have type 1 diabetes and are on a mixed-insulin regimen and note that your afternoon glucose reading is low on the days when you exercise in the morning, you and your physician may choose to increase your food intake or change the morning dose of your longer-acting insulin according to your activity level on those days.

Determining When to Check Your Blood Glucose

You need to know when you should monitor your blood sugar levels and what your glucose range should be. You and your health care team should determine this. It is generally recommended that you test your blood sugar just before you exercise, every 30 minutes during exercise, and 15 minutes after exercise. To prevent delayed-onset hypoglycemia, which typically occurs in the early stages of your exercise program or when the intensity of your activity increases, you should measure your glucose levels 6, 12, and 24 hours after cessation of exercise until your program has stabilized.

As a general guideline once your plan has stabilized, make sure that before exercising your glucose is at or slightly above 100 mg/dl. If your glucose is below 100 mg/dl, you should eat or drink something with carbohydrate in it until your blood glucose is in this range. The goal is to avoid hypoglycemia. If your glucose is at or above 100 mg/dl, then you need to take into account the effect that insulin or another glucose-lowering agent and exercise will have on your blood glucose, as discussed in detail in chapter 4. For instance, if you take insulin or have it in your system just before you exercise and you have not eaten, you are likely to experience a significant drop in your glucose level. Furthermore, it is generally accepted that exercise should be postponed if the glucose is more than 250 mg/dl and ketones are present in the urine, or if your glucose is greater than 300 mg/dl. (You can measure the urine ketone levels with urine test strips, which are available at your local pharmacy.) The American College of Sports Medicine (ACSM) guidelines state that if your glucose is between 200 and 400 mg/dl, you should consult your physician before exercising. If your glucose is greater than 400 mg/dl, the ACSM suggests that you do not exercise.

Glucose Too High to Exercise?

If your glucose is between 200 and 400 mg/dl, then you need medical supervision during exercise.
If your glucose is over 400 mg/dl, then seek medical attention and do not exercise.

Charting Weight Loss

In addition to glucose monitoring, weight control is important for those with type 2 diabetes. Charting your weight loss in your health diary can prove to be very rewarding. And this may be an interesting analysis of how exercise and diet can help you realize the positive changes described in this book. For instance, when comparing your weight against your average glucose over a three-month period, you are likely to see that your weight will decrease along with your average glucose level. You can compare your weight or glucose level to your heart rate, blood pressure, or laboratory values such as the hemoglobin A_{1C} as well. You can create charts similar to those in tables 7.1 and 7.2 to compare values.

The amount of weight you lose depends on your energy balance, as described in chapter 5. You and your health care team will develop a diet and exercise plan that you can incorporate into your lifestyle that will most likely allow you to lose an average of .5 to 2 pounds a week. As with most situations regarding your health, this will depend on your current activity level, physical abilities, and any other medical conditions. Furthermore, you are more likely to maintain long-term weight loss if you lose weight in smaller amounts over a longer time as opposed to losing large amounts of

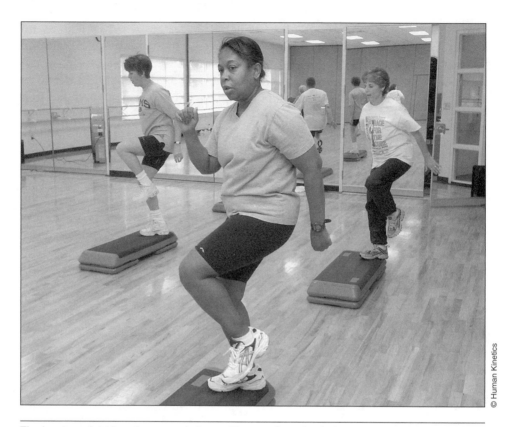

The key to weight loss is energy balance: The number of calories you burn must exceed the number of calories you take in.

weight over a short time. It is widely known that a dramatic weight loss in a short duration is largely due to body fluid loss and not to fat loss.

A good time to weigh yourself is in the morning, before you eat. Measuring your weight in this manner will give you more consistent results and less appearance of fluctuation in your weight over time. You should measure your weight a maximum of twice per week.

Responding to Change

When you start to see positive changes in your health, such as a decrease your weight or better control of your glucose, make sure that you document this in your health diary. The more pertinent information that you can record in an organized fashion in your diary (without obviously overdoing it), the easier it will be for you to find and capitalize on the key components that have allowed you some success. For example, if you have type 1 diabetes or type 2 diabetes requiring insulin, you may discover from your records that, on mornings when you exercise after taking your insulin, your glucose after breakfast is low. With this information you and your doctor can make the decision to decrease your rapid-acting insulin morning dose, change your exercising time, or change your meals.

If you have type 2 diabetes, you may find that your BMI has been decreasing, but you still have not achieved good glucose control. In this case you and your physician or dietitian may decide to analyze and make changes to the types of foods that you have been eating that may contribute to the elevated glucose levels. Or perhaps your physician will add glucose-lowering medication to your plan.

If you encounter a change in your health that would be considered negative, such as difficulty losing weight or symptoms of hypoglycemia or little or no change in weight, lipids, glucose levels, or blood pressure, document these results in your diary as well. In some cases it may be even more important to document the negative changes in comparison to the positive changes because some of these can pose a serious threat to your health.

If you find that you are not making progress in your action plan, it will be easier for you and your health care team to find solutions to the problems if your plan is well documented. For instance, you may find yourself gaining weight instead of losing weight while adhering to your action plan. This can be frustrating and may even cause you to quit your plan. Fortunately in most such cases, the problem and its solution lie within the realm of energy balance. It may be a simple miscalculation of the total number of calories you consume and the amount of exercise you need to burn those calories and create an energy deficit to stimulate weight loss. This is an easy problem to fix if you have detailed documentation of the intensity, duration, and type of exercise you are doing, along with the food log to allow you and your dietitian to redo the calculations to make your plan work for you. Sometimes the problem may be more difficult than this, but finding the solution will still be far easier if you have monitored and documented the details of what you have been doing in your action plan for diabetes.

You should note that you may not see a change in your weight for a couple weeks. Give your body some time to adjust the new activity and caloric intake. If you continue to have a problem despite recalculating your energy balance, visit your health care team for more specific guidance.

MONITORING PROGRESS AND RESPONDING TO CHANGE

☐ Start a health diary in a notebook, on your computer, or in another format that's convenient for you.

☐ Learn how to check your blood pressure at home.

☐ Make sure you are well-versed in how your particular method of glucose monitoring works, and know the best times to check and record glucose, especially with regard to exercise.

☐ Come up with a plan for keeping track of your weight. Perhaps devise a table in your health diary where you keep track of what you eat every day.

☐ Be aware of the changes that are happening in your body—both positive and negative—and have a plan for how you'll respond.

CHAPTER 8

TAKING MEDICATIONS AND SUPPLEMENTS

Throughout this book I have stressed the importance of understanding how diabetes affects you and how you can affect diabetes through exercise and healthy eating habits. In addition to prescribing exercise and a healthy diet, your doctor may add medications to your plan to optimize your glucose control. In this chapter we take a look at medications that can help you control your glucose levels and how exercise and diet may interact with those medications. In addition, we discuss the use of other medications and supplements that you may encounter and their potential effects on your health.

Drug Treatment of Type 1 Diabetes

People with type 1 diabetes use insulin to control their diabetes, and most use injections just underneath the skin (either via a hypodermic needle attached to a manual syringe or via an automatic delivery pump). Many with type 1 diabetes take a mixture of two types of insulin in the same injection. Typically one of the insulins has a rapid onset of action and a relatively short duration; the other insulin has a slower onset of action and a longer duration. This is referred to as a mixed dose. The most common form of rapid-acting, or short-acting, insulin is known as regular insulin. Another common short-acting insulin is called lispro (brand name is Humalog). Lispro is absorbed more rapidly than regular insulin, and it has a shorter duration. The most common longer-acting, or basal, insulin is called NPH insulin. Other types of longer-acting insulins may be used as well, such as lente, ultralente, and insulin glargine, which have very long durations of action and lower peak levels. Determining your correct insulin regimen can often be a process of trial and error. Your doctor will work with you and the other members of your health care team to determine the correct combinations and dosages of insulin for you.

As described previously, if you have type 1 diabetes you need to avoid hypoglycemia; you can accomplish this by taking great care to ensure that your carbohydrate and total caloric intake is coordinated with your insulin regimen. If you have type 1 diabetes and are exercising, it is even more important that your food intake and insulin dose correspond to the timing and amount of exercise you are doing. It is generally recommended that you do not exercise if your insulin's action is at or near its peak. It is best to exercise when your insulin's activity is low and your glucose levels are rising or higher than they are near the peak of your insulin's effectiveness. (See table 8.1.)

Table 8.1   Insulin Types and Durations

Insulin type	Onset (hours)	Peak (hours)	Duration (hours)
Regular (rapid-acting)	0.5-1	2-4	6-8
NPH (intermediate-acting)	1-3	6-12	18-26
Ultralente (long-acting)	4-8	12-18	24-28
Lantus (long-acting)	1	no pronounced peak	24

Monitoring your glucose regularly is critical to finding overall balance. Monitors have made individualized insulin modification simpler for patients and physicians. It is important to remember that each person's response will vary depending on the severity of the disease, exercise choice, and fitness level. A good starting point is decreasing the dose of short-acting insulin (regular or lispro) by 30 to 50 percent two to three hours before starting exercise. Those with an insulin pump may choose to decrease or eliminate the basal infusion of insulin during exercise. Many people with diabetes inject 1 to 3 units of regular or lispro insulin before exercise when their preexercise glucose levels are between 250 and 300 mg/dl (Colberg and Swain 2000). Keep in mind that hyperglycemia can cause dehydration; therefore, you should also monitor your hydration status.

If you have a significant amount of exercise or physical activity that is unplanned, be sure that you have some form of carbohydrate readily available to consume so that your blood glucose does not drop significantly and cause symptoms of hypoglycemia. You can typically prevent this by eating a snack before or during exercise.

The best way to avoid hypoglycemia is to discuss your specific exercise and diet plans with your health care team. Let your physician know about any changes you want to make in your diet and exercise plans so that he will be able to help you make adjustments to your insulin regimen that will help prevent hypoglycemia and control your glucose.

As discussed in chapter 7, it will also be beneficial for you to keep a detailed log of your insulin dose, food intake, and exercise intensity and duration while creating your action plan. Once your exercise routine and diet plan are stable, you can relax a little in your record keeping, but you still need to be aware of potential situations that can lead to hypoglycemia. You need to avoid hyperglycemia as well. You will typically run into this problem only if your insulin dose, caloric intake, and physical activity are not balanced.

Drugs on the Horizon

A new preparation of insulin is currently being tested that may allow insulin to be taken via an inhalation device such as those used by people with asthma. If these new delivery systems can consistently treat people with diabetes with the same or better safety and efficacy as insulin injections provide, then the advantage is clear—no more needle sticks from taking injections or disposing of needles. However, the disadvantages with this type of system are not as clear. For instance, how easy will it be to switch from your current injectable insulin to the inhaled form? Are there any long-term side effects from using inhaled insulin? Does exercise change the absorption rate of inhaled insulin? All these questions and many more have yet to be answered.

Drug Treatment of Type 2 Diabetes

If you have type 2 diabetes and are having a difficult time controlling your glucose with diet and exercise alone, your physician may decide to add a medication that will either increase your sensitivity to insulin, increase your production of insulin, or decrease the absorption of glucose from your gastrointestinal tract.

As discussed in chapter 1, people with type 2 diabetes typically have a decreased sensitivity to insulin. In other words, the insulin that is present in the body is not very effective at allowing glucose from the blood to pass into the cell. Medications that increase the sensitivity of the body's cells to insulin allow glucose to be used for energy by the cell by decreasing the level of blood glucose. Several forms of this medication, such as those referred to as biguanides, have a direct effect in the liver; other medications, commonly referred to as glitazones, have an effect predominantly in other tissues.

When glucose is high in the blood as a result of the cells' decreased sensitivity to insulin and the environment inside of each cell is low in glucose, the cells, particularly those in the liver, will begin a process called gluconeogenesis, which means a new generation of glucose. So even though the glucose is high in the blood, when the liver is insensitive to insulin it produces more glucose, which increases the glucose in the blood to an even higher level. The biguanides (Glucophage is a common brand name) increase the cells' sensitivity to insulin, thus allowing glucose to flow freely into the cell, which in turn decreases the glucose production in the liver. The glitazones (brand names Avandia and Actose) work similarly in other peripheral tissues.

The class of medication commonly used to treat type 2 diabetes increases the production of insulin in the pancreas. This type of medication is most effective in those with type 2 diabetes who have a lower production of insulin. The most common group in this class is referred to as sulfonylureas (some brand names are Amaryl, Diabeta, Diabinese, Dymelor, Glucotrol, Glynase, Micronase, Orinase, Tolinase). This type medication has been used for nearly half a century and has been improved, making it one of the most cost effective. Furthermore, because this type of medication increases your insulin levels, it is possible that you may experience hypoglycemia when taking them, especially when increasing your activity levels. Weight gain has also been associated with this class of medications. And again, to prevent hypoglycemia with exercise, you need to understand the symptoms and monitor your blood glucose levels when increasing your exercise duration or intensity. The newer drugs in this class of stimulators of insulin secretion (including Amaryl, Diabeta, Glucotrol, Glynase, and Micronase) have a quicker onset and a short duration, which may help lessen complications related to hypoglycemia and weight gain.

There is currently one other class of oral medication that can be used to decrease the blood glucose. These medications (acarbose, brand names Prandase and Precose; and miglitol, brand name Glyset) work by decreasing the absorption of carbohydrates from the gastrointestinal tract. The medications inhibit a crucial step in the breakdown of carbohydrates before they can be absorbed through the intestine into the bloodstream. However, because these medications need to be taken at the beginning of each meal, and common side effects are gas production and flatulence, these are used to a lesser extent than the three classes of drugs described previously.

People with type 2 diabetes who are having difficulty controlling glucose levels with exercise, diet, and one (or a combination) of oral medications may need to take insulin in a similar manner to those with type 1 diabetes. Frequent glucose monitoring is important here as well.

Other Medications and Supplements

You probably have encountered other medications or nutritional supplements at some time. Before starting your action plan for diabetes, meet with your physician to review all the medications or supplements that you are taking or that you plan on taking. There are several common medications that you may use for conditions other than diabetes, which may increase or decrease your blood glucose levels (see table 8.2). In addition, you may wish to use nutritional or ergogenic supplements to enhance your overall program. With the exception of the two supplements chromium and creatine (which I discuss later), I will not talk about supplements specifically.

Table 8.2   *Common Medications That May Affect Blood Glucose*

May decrease blood glucose levels	May increase blood glucose levels
Blood pressure medications:	**Blood pressure medications:**
alpha-blockers: prazosin, terazosin, doxazosin;	**diuretics (water pills):** hydrochlorothiazide, furosemide, metolazone;
ACE inhibitors: quinapril, ramipril, enalapril;	**beta-blockers:** atenolol, propranolol, metoprolol;
beta-blockers: atenolol, propranolol, metoprolol	**calcium channel blockers (dihydropyridines):** nifedipine, nicardipine, amlodipine
Salicylates: aspirin, diflunisal, salsalate	**Glucocorticoids:** cortisone, prednisone, methylprednisolone
Alcohol	**Niacin**

Adapted, by permission, from Neil Ruderman and John T. Devlin, 1995, *The health professional's guide to diabetes and exercise* (Alexandria, VA: American Diabetes Association), 236.

Many supplements are available that may or may not be as effective as their labels claim. In addition, many of the supplements have not been investigated thoroughly enough to allow manufacturers to make truthful or accurate claims; this can pose a danger to anyone taking them. But more important, if you were to take a supplement and there was an unanticipated effect on the blood glucose level, it could result in a significant problem with your action plan for diabetes. My personal stance on nutritional supplement use (other than multiple vitamins) in people with diabetes is that their use should be discouraged until we have more definitive information about their effects on glucose control. However, as more data become available, supplements may have a place in the treatment of diabetes. With further research, the following supplements may prove to be of some benefit to people with diabetes.

Chromium Picolinate

Chromium picolinate (the most popular form of chromium) is a trace mineral found in the human body that is required for carbohydrate and

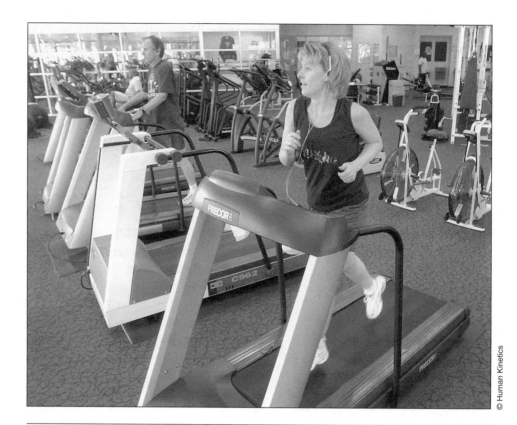

Before going full-steam into your exercise program, it's crucial to know if your medication has any interactions with exercise.

fat metabolism. It is thought that chromium helps insulin bind to the cells' receptors, thus enhancing insulin sensitivity. In fact, some researchers have reported significant decreases in hemoglobin A_{1C} and total cholesterol values in those with type 2 diabetes who supplement with 500 micrograms of chromium picolinate (a higher dose than the estimated safe and adequate daily dietary intake [ESADDI] of 50 to 200 micrograms) (Anderson et al. 1997). In addition, multiple studies have shown that chromium supplementation does not increase body mass, strength, or muscle size as once thought. However, another study has shown that people who were taking chromium lost significantly more body weight and fat than those on similar diet plans who were not taking chromium (Kaats et al. 1996). Recognize that we need more research in these areas to generate sufficient evidence before we can make the statement that chromium picolinate is safe and effective in treating diabetes.

Creatine

Creatine is a popular nutritional supplement used in the amateur and professional fitness world. It is a substance made in the liver, pancreas, and kidneys, but it can also be acquired from eating meats and fish. Creatine has been shown to increase muscle strength and muscle size as well as increase fat-free (lean) mass in conjunction with strength training (Becque et al. 2000). Interestingly, researchers have reported that creatine may facilitate the removal of glucose from the blood and may reduce gluconeogenesis (new production of glucose) in the liver in people with type 1 diabetes who have high blood glucose levels (Rocic et al. 1991). As with all supplements, much more definitive research needs to be done on creatine and glucose control before its use can be recommended in people with diabetes.

The study of nutritional supplements is a very active field, and many of the data available do not pertain to the enhancement of the treatment of diabetes. Thus, I do not recommend using any supplements without the guidance of your health care team, especially in the initial phases of your plan when you are vulnerable to other problems. At this point I do not encourage supplement use in my patients with diabetes because of lack of evidence of their safety or efficacy.

Whether you take a medication to control your glucose or are contemplating adding a supplement to your diet, you should now have some understanding of how these substances may affect your health. Keep abreast of changes in medications that you are currently taking and the development of new ones, and check with your doctor before making any changes to your diabetes treatment. These steps will help you stay on top of your action plan.

ACTION PLAN:
TAKING MEDICATIONS AND SUPPLEMENTS

☐ Know which medications are available for your type of diabetes, and research those medications further, especially if you are taking one.

☐ Talk to your doctor about how your medication may be affected by changes in exercise or diet. This should be done before making any changes.

☐ Be aware of the possible side effects of the medication you are taking and how to avoid or deal with them.

☐ Consider and talk to your doctor about the possible use of supplements, but do not proceed with use until you've carefully and thoroughly researched the options. Know the pros, cons, and risks of each one.

CHAPTER 9

MAINTAINING LONG-TERM CONTROL

Now that you are well underway in your action plan for diabetes, we will discuss ways of maintaining your success. You have set short-term goals that have been linked together to meet your main goal of glucose control through an active and healthy lifestyle. Your challenge now is to reeducate yourself about diabetes as new knowledge is gained in this field and to keep up with new technology. With this newly gained knowledge and technology, you must remotivate yourself to make the necessary changes to your action plan and promise yourself that you will keep on moving forward.

In chapter 7 we discussed ways to monitor your progress and how to respond to change. The same principles carry over into the maintenance phase of your action plan. It will be important for you to meet with your health care team at least once a year during the maintenance phase and more frequently (every three months) in the earlier phases to ensure that you are on track. New information may become available that your physician will be aware of and can pass on to you. But more important, your health care team will be available for you as challenges present themselves. They can help you make the correct changes in response to these problems and to avoid potential frustrations.

You must understand what the common complications are and how to avoid them. It is even more important to understand what to do if you are faced with them. As we discussed in chapter 3, just as the lead planner of the project to send a spaceship to Mars and back to Earth has to be prepared for all situations, you have to be prepared to deal with potential problems and have a rescue plan in place. The best way to create your rescue plan is to identify the things that may interrupt your exercise plans or interfere with your healthy eating habits. For instance, say you find yourself skipping exercise sessions to watch television. Or say that you find yourself going out with friends and indulging in high-calorie foods several times a week. The best preventive measure is to recognize the triggers early and have a rescue plan in place. Let's look at some sample situations and ways of dealing with them.

Decreased Exercise

You may find yourself exercising less than you had planned. This may come about for several reasons: illness, work, school, family obligations, moving, vacations, and so on. Whatever the issue may be, you need a plan so that you can preempt a relapse into your old habits. Say you were sick for one week and were unable to exercise. The solution to this problem could be as simple as setting a realistic and reasonable restart date on

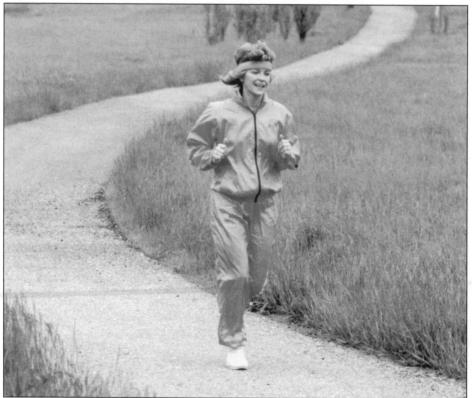

© Jim Whitmer

Bumps along the road are inevitable, but a good action plan and strategies for motivation will keep you on track and reaping the benefits of a healthy lifestyle.

the calendar, such as 10 days from the start of your illness, and having a friend, family member, or exercise partner give you a reminder. If you recover from your illness sooner than expected, then start back earlier. Remember to start at a comfortable pace until you are back on track. A reasonable time frame to be back on track after resuming your plan is around two weeks. However, if your illness lasts longer than a week or if you have had a severe illness such as influenza, which can involve significant fluid loss from diarrhea and vomiting, you should see your physician before restarting your program.

You can also set a restart date if you have special work-related circumstances, moving days, or vacations that pull you away from exercise. But most situations in life allow time for some exercise and, as discussed in chapter 4, splitting your exercise routine up into smaller, more manageable sessions is still effective. However, for those situations that do not allow for split exercise sessions, you need to recognize when your exercise decreases so that you can resume your plan as soon as possible.

Another strategy is to enlist the help of another person. For example, have a friend keep an envelope of your money. Your friend is not to return your money until you restart your program. You can even notify your health care team that you are unable to exercise for a short time, and then ask them if they could call you with a reminder to restart your program.

No matter what method you use to prevent the relapse into an unhealthy lifestyle, your main focus should be to keep on track with your program. Whether splitting up your exercise routines into smaller, more manageable sessions for a short time or stopping exercise for a week with a planned restart date, you must not allow yourself to fall back into an unhealthy lifestyle. The longer you are away from exercise, the more likely you are to slip back into your old habits and the more difficult it will be to regain the success you have achieved. From my own experience, you will find it easier to get back into your program if you do not miss more than three consecutive days of exercise.

Sample Rescue Plans for Decreased Exercise

▷ Set a realistic and reasonable restart date as soon as you stop exercising, and have friends, family members, or exercise partners call to remind you.

▷ Temporarily split up your exercise sessions into shorter ones to make them more manageable during difficult times.

▷ Place some money in an envelope and give it to a friend; ask your friend to return the money to you *only* when you resume your program.

Increased Caloric Consumption

Relapsing into old eating habits may be one of the most difficult problems to overcome in the first year of an action plan for diabetes. In thinking about this, recognize what situations may trigger you to overeat. Eating for most people is a social event. Most of us have lunch dates with colleagues or friends on a weekly or even daily basis. At this point you have likely made changes to your eating habits that are more conducive to your goal of glucose control. But it is important to be aware that falling into old habits may be easier than you anticipate. For instance, you may have made changes in your diet and have been eating healthier foods, but one day you decide to meet friends at a restaurant that is known for serving mostly deep-fried foods. You may decide not to be the "odd guy out," and you have your share of high-calorie food—not to mention that this kind of food tastes unbelievably good! Doing so does not qualify as a relapse. But making this a regular part of your life certainly does.

So where should you draw the line? The best way to do this is to calculate your caloric intake versus your calories burned with exercise, and then balance this out, as discussed in chapter 5. For example, if you decide to eat a not-so-healthy meal, estimate the number of calories you've eaten over your planned calories, and increase your exercise to burn off those calories over a one- to four-day period. So if you ate an estimated 1,000 extra calories in a day, you should burn an extra 1,000 calories over that week. Split up the extra exercise into three or four days to burn an extra 333 calories each day for three days, or 250 calories each day for four days. But be aware that doing this even as infrequently as once per week can lead to regression toward your old lifestyle. Calories have a way of adding up faster than you might think! Having an occasional higher-calorie meal followed by a planned increase in exercise will allow you to have some balance in your life, but I would recommend this only once your plan has been stabilized and no more frequently than twice per month. Even so, I would not encourage you to plan these types of meals in your diet on a regular basis.

Sample Rescue Plan for Increased Caloric Consumption

▷ Estimate the amount of calories over your planned calories and increase your exercise to burn off those calories over a three- to four-day period.

▷ Be aware that doing this even as infrequently as once per week can lead to regression toward your old lifestyle.

Contracts

If you find yourself falling into the trap of relapse, devising a contract with your health care team may help. The contract is an agreement between you and your health care team that is designed to help you keep on track. The details of this contract will depend on what you can anticipate as being problems for you, and your contract must be realistic in order to work. For instance, you may have a contract with your health care team that says that you will lose three to four pounds per month until you reach your goal (see sample contract in figure 9.1). Or you may have a contract that states that you progress at a certain rate in your exercise program until you reach your goal. You can incorporate many things into a contract, but you must understand that you're doing this for your own benefit. The only person who will suffer from a breach of contract will be you. Your health care team will be flexible, understanding that your needs and desires may change; they will respond to that in kind, ensuring that you meet your goals.

SAMPLE CONTRACT

I, John Doe, promise to myself and my health care team that I will adhere to my action plan of losing 3 pounds per month until I reach my goal weight of 165 pounds. If, for reasons beyond my control (such as an illness or significant personal or family issue), I am unable to adhere to my program for more than three consecutive days, I will immediately put my rescue plan into action.

X_____

John Doe

Figure 9.1 Sample contract.

The keys to maintaining your success are largely dependent on your understanding of your personal health goals. In this book I have defined the types of diabetes and explained how diabetes can affect you as well as how exercise affects diabetes. I've discussed nutritional components crucial to good health and how to develop a healthy lifestyle. You have put these together to create a personalized plan that supports the primary goal of glucose control. I wish you the best success. Remember that you must reeducate, remotivate, and keep moving!

MAINTAINING LONG-TERM CONTROL

☐ Anticipate the problems that could occur that would pull you off track with your action plan.

- Illness or injury
- Travel
- Events that disturb your usual schedule
- Increase in caloric intake

☐ Make a contingency plan for all of these situations so that if they happen, you can minimize the disturbance to your plan.

☐ Find friends who will help you stay committed through encouragement and motivation.

REFERENCES

Anderson, R.A., N. Cheng, and N.A. Bryden. 1997. Elevated intakes of supplemental chromium improve glucose and insulin variables in individuals with type 2 diabetes. *Diabetes* 46(110):1786-1791.

Artal, R. 1996. Exercise: An alternative therapy for gestational diabetes. *The Physician and Sports Medicine* 24(3):54-66.

Becque, M.D., J.D. Lochmann, and D.R. Melrose. 2000. Effects of oral creatine supplementation on muscular strength and body composition. *Medicine and Science in Sports and Exercise* 32(3):654-658.

Brooks, G., and J. Mercer. 1994. The balance of carbohydrate and lipid utilization during exercise: The "crossover" concept. *Journal of Applied Physiology* 16(4):635-662.

Colberg, S.R., and D.P. Swain. 2000. Exercise and diabetes control. *The Physician and Sports Medicine* 28(8):63-81.

DeFronzo, R.A. 1988. Lilly Lecture. The Triumvirate: Beta cell, muscle, liver. A collusion responsible for NIDDM. *Diabetes* 37:667-687.

Devlin, J. 1992. Effects of exercise on insulin sensitivity in humans. *Diabetes Care* 15(11):1690-1693.

Harris, M.I., K.M. Flegal, C.C. Cowie, M.S. Eberhardt, D.E. Goldstein, R.R. Little, H.M. Wiedmeyer, and D.D. Byrd-Holt. 1994. Prevalence of diabetes, impaired fasting glucose, and impaired glucose tolerance in U.S. adults. The Third National Health and Nutrition Examination Survey. *Diabetes Care* 21(4):518-524.

Hostetter, T.H. 2003. Prevention of the development and progression of renal disease. *Journal of the American Society of Nephrology* 14(7): S144-147.

Hu, F.B., R.J. Sigal, J.W. Rich-Edwards, G.A. Colditz, C.G. Solomon, W.C. Willett, F.E. Speizer, and J.E. Manson. 1999. Walking compared with vigorous physical activity and risk of type 2 diabetes in women: A prospective study. *Journal of the American Medical Association* 282(15): 1433-1439.

Kaats, G.R., K. Blum, J.A. Fisher, and J.A. Adelman. 1996. Effects of chromium picolinate supplementation on body composition: A randomized, double-masked, placebo-controlled study. *Current Therapeutic Research* 57:747-756.

Laaksonen, D.E., M. Atalay, L.K. Niskanen, J. Mustonen, C.K. Sen, and T.A. Lakka. 2000. Aerobic exercise and the lipid profile in type 1 diabetic men: A randomized controlled trial. *Medicine and Science in Sports and Exercise* 32(9):1541-1548.

Larsen, P.R. 2003. Pharmacotherapy of type 2 diabetes. In R. Hardin Williams (ed.) *Williams Textbook of Endocrinology* (10th ed). Philadelphia: Elsevier.

Lee, I.M., K.M. Rexrode, N.R. Cook, J.E. Manson, and J.E. Buring. 2001. Physical activity and coronary heart disease in women: Is "no pain, no gain" passé? *Journal of the American Medical Association* 285:1447-1454.

Manson, J.E., E.B. Rimm, M.J. Stampfer, G.A. Colditz, W.C. Willett, A.S. Krolewski, B. Rosner, C.H. Hennekens, and F.E. Speizer. 1991. A prospective study of physical activity and incidence of noninsulin-dependent diabetes mellitus in women. *Lancet* 338:774-778.

Marshall, J., S. Hoag, S. Shetterly, and R. Hamman. 1994. Dietary fat predicts conversion from impaired glucose tolerance to NIDDM. The San Luis Valley Diabetes Study. *Diabetes Care* 17:50-56.

McArdle, W.D., F.I. Katch, and V.L. Katch. 2000. *Essential of exercise physiology* (2nd ed). Baltimore: Lippincott William & Wilkins.

Mokdad, A.H., E.S. Ford, B.A. Bowman, W.H. Dietz, F. Vinicor, V.S. Bales, and J.S. Marks. 2003. Prevalence of obesity, diabetes, and obesity-related health risk factors. *Journal of the American Medical Association* 289(1):76-79.

Raben, A., J.J. Holst, J. Madsen, and A. Astrup. 1994. Resistant starch: The effect on postprandial glycemia, hormonal response, and satiety. *American Journal of Clinical Nutrition* 60:544-551.

Rocic, B., D. Breyer, M. Granic, and S. Milutinovic. 1991. The effect of guanidine substances from uremic plasma on insulin binding to erythrocyte receptors in uremia. *Hormone and Metabolic Research* 23(10):490-494.

Rocic, B., Z. Turk, I. Misur, and M. Vucic. 1995. Effect of creatine on glycation of albumin in vitro. *Hormone and Metabolic Research* 27(11): 511-512.

Swinburn B.A., P.A. Metcalf, and S.J. Ley. 2001. Long-term (5 year) effects of a reduced-fat diet intervention in individuals with glucose intolerance. *Diabetes Care* 24:619-624.

Turok, D.K., S.D. Ratcliffe, and E.G. Baxely. 2003. Management of gestational diabetes mellitus. *American Family Physician* 68(9):1767-1772.

Wee, C.C., E.P. McCarthy, R.B. Davis, and R.S. Phillips. 1999. Physician counseling about exercise. *Journal of the American Medical Association* 282:1583-1588.

White R.D., and C. Sherman. 1999. Exercise in diabetes management. *The Physician and Sports Medicine* 4(27):63-76.

INDEX

Note: The italicized *f* and *t* following page numbers refer to figures and tables, respectively.

ABOUT THE AUTHOR

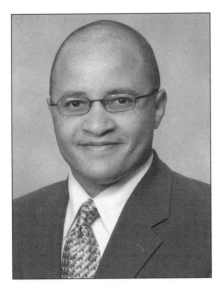

Darryl E. Barnes, **MD,** is a consultant and instructor with the department of family medicine and musculoskeletal clinic at the Mayo Clinic in Rochester, Minnesota. He specializes in total care of physically active people, including those with diabetes. He is a family physician with certified added qualifications (CAQ) in primary care sports medicine and is the team physician for all teams at Rochester Community Technical College and for the Rochester Giants, a U.S. semiprofessional football team.

Dr. Barnes has lectured on diabetes, nutrition, and athletics on behalf of the Mayo Clinic and was on the medical staff for the 25th Ironman Triathlon World Championship in 2003. He is a member of the American College of Sports Medicine, the American Medical Society for Sports Medicine, the American Academy of Family Physicians, the American Medical Association, and the Performing Arts Medicine Association.

Dr. Barnes lives in Rochester, Minnesota, with his wife, Aimee. He enjoys running, fishing, and playing golf in his spare time.

ABOUT THE ACSM

The **American College of Sports Medicine (ACSM)** is more than the world's leader in the scientific and medical aspects of sports and exercise; it is an association of people and professions exploring the use of medicine and exercise to make life healthier for all people.

Since 1954, ACSM has been committed to the promotion of physical activity and the diagnosis, treatment, and prevention of sports-related injuries. With more than 20,000 international, national, and regional chapter members in 80 countries, ACSM is internationally known as the leading source of state-of-the-art research and information on sports medicine and exercise science. Through ACSM, health and fitness professionals representing a variety of disciplines work to improve the quality of life for people around the world through health and fitness research, education, and advocacy.

A large part of ACSM's mission is devoted to public awareness and education about the positive aspects of physical activity for people of all ages, from all walks of life. ACSM's physicians, researchers, and educators have created tools to help people lead healthier lives—whether they're looking to start an exercise program or avoid and treat sports injuries.

ACSM's National Center is located in Indianapolis, Indiana, widely recognized as the amateur sports capitol of the nation. Contact ACSM by phone at 317-637-9200, or visit the Web site at www.acsm.org for detailed department and staff information and facts on health and fitness, nutrition, sport-specific training and injuries, and more.

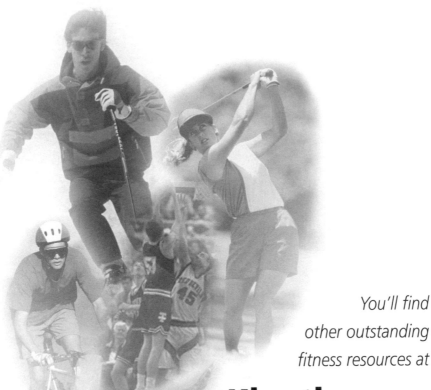